Caregiving with Pride

T0251498

Caregiving with Pride has been co-published simultaneously as *Journal of Gay & Lesbian Social Services*, Volume 18, Numbers 3/4 2007.

Caregiving with Pride

Karen I. Fredriksen-Goldsen, PhD
Editor

Caregiving with Pride has been co-published simultaneously as *Journal of Gay & Lesbian Social Services*, Volume 18, Numbers 3/4 2007.

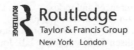

Routledge
Taylor & Francis Group
New York   London

First published by The Haworth Press, Inc.

10 Industrial Avenue, Mahwah, New Jersey 07430

This edition published 2012 by Routledge

Routledge
Taylor & Francis Group
711 Third Avenue
New York, NY 10017

Routledge
Taylor & Francis Group
2 Park Square, Milton Park
Abingdon, Oxon OX14 4RN

Caregiving with Pride has been co-published simultaneously as *Journal of Gay & Lesbian Social Services*, Volume 18, Numbers 3/4 2007.

The development, preparation, and publication of this work has been undertaken with great care. However, the publisher, employees, editors, and agents of The Haworth Press and all imprints of The Haworth Press, Inc., including The Haworth Medical Press® and Pharmaceutical Products Press®, are not responsible for any errors contained herein or for consequences that may ensue from use of materials or information contained in this work. With regard to case studies, identities and circumstances of individuals discussed herein have been changed to protect confidentiality. Any resemblance to actual persons, living or dead, is entirely coincidental.

The Haworth Press is committed to the dissemination of ideas and information according to the highest standards of intellectual freedom and the free exchange of ideas. Statements made and opinions expressed in this publication do not necessarily reflect the views of the Publisher, Directors, management, or staff of The Haworth Press, Inc., or an endorsement by them.

Library of Congress Cataloging-in-Publication Data

Caregiving with pride / Karen I. Fredriksen-Goldsen, editor.
     p. cm.
     "Co-published simultaneously as Journal of gay & lesbian social services, volume 18, numbers 3/4 2007."
     Includes bibliographical references and index.
     ISBN-13: 978-1-56023-759-4 (soft cover : alk. paper)
     1. Gays–Social conditions. 2. Gays–Services for. 3. Gay caregivers. 4. Care of the sick. 5. Social work with gays. I. Fredriksen-Goldsen, Karen I. II. Journal of gay & lesbian social services.
HQ76.25.C36 2007
362'.0425–dc22

2007035096

ABOUT THE EDITOR

Karen I. Fredriksen-Goldsen, PhD, is the Director of the Institute for Multigenerational Health, the Associate Dean for Academic Affairs and an Associate Professor at the University of Washington, School of Social Work. Dr. Fredriksen-Goldsen is a leading expert on caregiving, multigenerational practice, and family care within diverse and marginalized communities. Her research has been nationally recognized and she is the principal investigator on several funded research projects that examine the needs and experiences of informal caregivers and care receivers across diverse communities. She conducted the first national survey of caregiving responsibilities within gay and lesbian communities and completed one of the first studies on HIV/AIDS caregivers and care recipient partnerships. Currently, she is an investigator on a project to design and test an HIV antiretroviral adherence project in China, utilizing family caregivers for an intervention component. She is also the principal investigator of a project funded by the Hartford Foundation that examines the needs and experiences of caregiving partners in historically disadvantaged communities. Her book, *Families and Work: New Directions in the Twenty-First Century,* published by Oxford University Press, has been well received as the most comprehensive study to date of caregiving across the lifespan. She and colleagues recently published a book, *Looking Back, Looking Forward: The Lives of Lesbian Elders,* which examines resilience within a historical context and addresses important life transitions, including aging, identity development, adversity and family life.

Dr. Fredriksen-Goldsen received the Outstanding Research Award by the Society for Social Work and Research and was selected as a Hartford Geriatric Social Work Faculty Scholar by the John A. Hartford Foundation and the Gerontological Society of America. Locally, nationally and internationally, Dr. Fredriksen-Goldsen has provided consultation and training on caregiving and multigenerational practice across the lifespan. She received her PhD in Social Welfare from the University of California at Berkeley.

Caregiving with Pride

CONTENTS

About the Contributors

David W. Coon, PhD, is a faculty member at Arizona State University's Department of Social and Behavioral Sciences. Previously, Dr. Coon served as the Associate Director of the Older Adult & Family Center of the VA Palo Alto Health Care System and Stanford University School of Medicine and Research Scientist at UCSF/Mt. Zion Institute on Aging in San Francisco. He has authored or coauthored over 70 journal articles, books chapters, monographs and treatment manuals, and has been instrumental in the development and implementation of successful community-based and university based programs serving diverse populations for over 15 years. Dr. Coon currently coordinates a number of research programs in family caregiving, including LGBT caregiving issues, HIV over 50, and longevity.

Anthony R. D'Augelli, PhD, is Associate Dean for Undergraduate Studies and Outreach in the College of Health and Human Development at Penn State University. He is a faculty member in the Department of Human Development and Family Studies, in which he is Professor of Human Development. Dr. D'Augelli has conducted numerous research projects on different aspects of sexual orientation development over the lifespan, most recently a longitudinal study of the impact of antigay victimization on the mental health of lesbian, gay, and bisexual youth.

Eliza A. Dragowski, PhD, is Substitute Assistant Professor in the graduate programs of school psychology and school counseling of the Education Department at Brooklyn College of the City University of New York. She received her doctorate from the School Psychology Program in The Steinhardt School of Culture, Education, and Human Development at New York University.

Teresa (Tessa) Evans-Campbell, PhD, is Assistant Professor at the University of Washington (UW) School of Social Work (SSW). She directs the Institute for Indigenous Health and Child Welfare Research and researches the effects of historical trauma, including boarding school experience, on indigenous families. Dr. Evans-Campbell is an enrolled citizen of the Snohomish Tribes of Indians.

Karen I. Fredriksen-Goldsen, PhD, is Associate Dean for Academic Affairs and the Director of the Institute for Multigenerational Health, Development, and Equality at the University of Washington, School of Social Work. She is the recipient of the Outstanding Research Award by the Society for Social Work and Research and is the Principal Investigator on several funded research projects. Dr. Fredriksen-Goldsen has published extensively on caregiving, work and family, family care within marginalized populations, and multigenerational practice. She is the author of the book, *Families and Work: New Directions in the Twenty-First Century*, published by Oxford University Press.

Pat A. Freeman, PhD, is actively involved with the Northwest LGBT History Project. He has done numerous presentations on gay/lesbian history for universities, high schools, and community organizations. Since his female-to-male (FTM) transition, Dr. Freeman has shifted his focus to include transgender issues.

Arnold H. Grossman, PhD, is Professor and Associate Chair of the Department of Applied Psychology, The Steinhardt School of Culture, Education, and Human Development at New York University (NYU). His teaching, research and service focus on people who experience stigmatization and marginalization, primarily the development and mental health of lesbian, gay, bisexual, and transgender (LGBT) youth and the physical and mental health of older LGB adults. He has been a research investigator on numerous studies related to these populations.

Nancy R. Hooyman, PhD, is the Hooyman Professor in Gerontology and Dean Emeritus at the University of Washington, School of Social Work, and co-director of the School's Institute for Multigenerational Health Development and Equality. She is co-Principal Investigator of the John A. Hartford-funded CSWE National Center on Gerontological Social Work Education, co-PI of the Hartford Planning Grant National Center for Family Care Initiatives, and PI of the Hartford Practicum Partnership Project at the School of Social Work. She is author of eleven books and over 100 articles and chapters related to gerontology and women's issues and is a frequent presenter at conferences on gerontology, older women, end-of-life care, caregiving, and gerontological curricular change.

Charles P. Hoy-Ellis (formerly Charles W. Ellis), MSW, is a Chemical Dependency Counselor, HIV-Specialist, Mental Health Therapist, and Case Manager at Seattle Counseling Service for Sexual Minorities. He works primarily with gay and bisexual men who are living with HIV/AIDS, substance abuse and mental health issues. He received his Master of Social Work (clinical) degree from the University of Washington. His research has included personality and ego-development, and the meaning, experience and context of gay and bisexual men living with HIV/AIDS. He has presented his research at regional and international conferences and is a recipient of the *Jane Loevinger Award for Excellence in Research.*

R. Andrew Shippy, PhC, is a Senior Research Associate at ACRIA, where he is the Principal Investigator of the ROAH Program, a cohort study of 1,000 HIV-positive adults over age 50. His primary research interests include the effects of chronic illness and stigma on social support and psychological well-being among vulnerable populations, including elders with vision impairment, LGBT seniors, and older adults living with HIV.

Antony Stately, PhD, is Project Director of the HONOR Project, a research project exploring health and wellness among two-spirit people, and directs the Center for Translational and Implementation Research and Dissemination at the University of Washington. He is Oenida and Ojibwe.

Karina L. Walters, PhD, holds the William P. and Ruth Gerberding University Professorship at the University of Washington, School of Social Work. She is Director of the Institute for Indigenous Wellness Research and conducts research on cultural strengths in indigenous populations that buffer the effect of historical trauma and discrimination on health. Dr. Walters is an enrolled citizen of the Choctaw Nation of Oklahoma.

Mark E. Williams, MSW, MDiv, is a grief counselor at Providence Hospice of Seattle and a research assistant with the Relationship Research Institute. He serves as chairperson of the Community Advisory Board for MPowerment, a queer youth empowerment project in Seattle, and an advocate and community organizer for lesbian, gay, bisexual and transgender rights within religious communities.

Preface

As in most societies worldwide, the population of the United States is aging dramatically. The majority of elders in industrialized societies with well-developed public health care and inclusive health care financing systems are enjoying good health and high functioning longer. However, with increasing age comes an increased likelihood of need for help from others. Most of the assistance elders and other disabled adults need is provided by friends and by family members, alone or in partnership with health and social service agencies. In the United States, gerontology has long recognized that attention to this informal system of care is essential, but when it comes to aging among gay and lesbian people, the topic of caregiving is quite new. However, the unpaid work of kin and non-kin is also vital to the well-being of children and of ill or disabled adults as well, as the HIV epidemic has so memorably demonstrated in many gay communities in the United States.

This ground-breaking volume provides a comprehensive examination of gay, lesbian, bisexual and transgender (GLBT) caregiving, with a glimpse of issues involved in needing or receiving care as well. Editor Karen Fredriksen-Goldsen, a leading expert and nationally-known researcher on caregiving in marginalized communities and multigenerational relationships, has collected and commissioned articles that address a range of LGBT caregiving issues comprehensively and creatively. Many articles provide summaries and analyses of the literature in various areas related to LGBT caregiving. Others include reports of original research. The volume reflects a biopsychosocial perspective, which is necessary to understanding the varied aspects of this topic. The articles both insist on and illustrate the importance of taking both identity issues, espe-

[Haworth co-indexing entry note]: "Preface." Anastas, Jeane W. Co-published simultaneously in *Journal of Gay & Lesbian Social Services* (The Haworth Press, Inc.) Vol. 18, No. 3/4, 2007, pp. xxv-xxvii; and: *Caregiving with Pride* (ed: Karen I. Fredriksen-Goldsen) The Haworth Press, Inc., 2007, pp. xix-xxi. Single or multiple copies of this article are available for a fee from The Haworth Document Delivery Service [1-800-HAWORTH, 9:00 a.m. - 5:00 p.m. (EST). E-mail address: docdelivery@haworthpress.com].

cially but not only issues of sexual orientation and gender expression, and the social, cultural, and policy contexts of caregiving into account. Taken together, the papers address health issues and needs of those needing care, including the impact of HIV; the psychological effects, positive and negative, of caregiving; family and personal ("chosen family") relationships; interactions with formal systems of health and long-term care; the effects of history and social stigma on those who need care and those who give it; and how current social policies impede LGBT people in their access to care and LGBT caregivers in their efforts to help. Looking closely at the situations of transgender people reminds us that there are special health risks that transgender (and gay, lesbian, and bisexual people) face. Listening to the voices of two-spirit people who are caregivers opens up possibilities for re-framing and re-claiming the positives in giving care and for re-emphasizing the community-wide contributions of LGBT caregiving in all of its forms.

Because caregiving issues, for LGBT caregivers and LGBT care recipients, span so many areas yet have so far been overlooked, much more research is needed, a point made most strongly in the concluding article of this collection. This article and this volume call out for new ways of conceptualizing caregiving research, such as recognizing its dyadic nature and the different meanings given to caregiving in different cultural and ethnic groups, and for new research methodologies, including ways of recruiting more representative and more diverse samples from within what can be "hidden" communities. Most important, the authors call for questioning and challenging our current service delivery systems, in aging, health care, chronic and long-term care, and child care, and our current health, housing, employment, and social insurance policies until we can be confident that all LGBT people needing care and all LGBT people giving care are equitably treated.

The first step, however, is to put LGBT caregiving "on the map," because the care that LGBT people provide within their families of origin, to their partners, within their friendship networks, and within their communities as a whole should be indeed a source of pride. Celebrating this form of generativity once again belies the myth that LGBT people are affluent self-involved "singles" uninvolved in family and community life (Anastas, 2001). This volume begins to tell this special story of "caregiving with pride" in many of its varieties. It will be a valuable resource for research and scholarship to come. It will also be essential reading for those concerned with the present and the future development of health and social services to meet the needs of all of those LGBT people who may now or one day need care, and for all of those LGBT people who give care, that is, for all of us.

Jeane W. Anastas, Editor
Journal of Gay & Lesbian Social Services

REFERENCE

Anastas, J. W. (2001). Economic rights, economic myths, and economic realities. *Journal of Gay & Lesbian Social Services, 13* (1/2), 99-116. Simultaneously published as a chapter in *From hate crimes to human rights: A tribute to Matthew Shepard*, pp. 99-116, M. E. Swigonski, R. S. Mama, & K. Ward, Eds. Binghamton, NY: Harrington Park Press.

Caregiving with Pride:
An Introduction

Karen I. Fredriksen-Goldsen
Charles P. Hoy-Ellis

*Oh, boy. I would say there would be times that I was absolutely terrified
and she would still be there, and that could be as simple as trying to
take a bath. And, she always managed to pull it off.*

*I mean there's things that have been particularly important—
he had a problem a few years ago where he was passing out
and I ended up taking him to the hospital and he actually
had to get a pacemaker. So that was actually a very stressful time,
but it was something we got through.*

*Well, she fell out of bed, broke both of her feet, we called 911
and they came. They weren't paying attention to what I was saying.
And it was sort of a nightmare that time. It gets very bad
when in a period of a week she's got so many conditions that
there will be a crisis with this condition, a crisis with that condition, like
three different urgent things and I'm trying to be with her in some way with
all of them, and it's just absolutely exhausting.*

*And I had kind of hit the wall in terms of my pain level and
energy level. So after that point I was like—he must really love [me].*

[Haworth co-indexing entry note]: "Caregiving with Pride: An Introduction." Fredriksen-Goldsen, Karen
I., and Charles P. Hoy-Ellis. Co-published simultaneously in *Journal of Gay & Lesbian Social Services* (The
Haworth Press, Inc.) Vol. 18, No. 3/4, 2007, pp. 1-13; and: *Caregiving with Pride* (ed: Karen I. Fredriksen-
Goldsen) The Haworth Press, Inc., 2007, pp. 1-13. Single or multiple copies of this article are available for a
fee from The Haworth Document Delivery Service [1-800-HAWORTH, 9:00 a.m. - 5:00 p.m. (EST). E-mail
address: docdelivery@haworthpress.com].

doi:10.1300/J041v18n03_01

INTRODUCTION

Family members and friends are the primary caregivers in this country, providing the majority of assistance to ill and disabled persons when needed. It is more common now than ever before for partners, family members and friends to provide informal care because of the aging of the population and the trend toward noninstitutional care. Yet, caregiving in LGBT (lesbian, gay, bisexual and transgender) communities has received insufficient attention, even though informal caregiving across diverse communities is the backbone of our long-term care system.

Caregiving is defined here as unpaid assistance, provided primarily by family members, friends and neighbors, to help individuals remain in the community. The significant increase in the older population and the trend toward noninstitutional care are significantly altering caregiving in this country. Most long-term care for adults age 65 and over is provided not in nursing homes but informally and privately, at little or no public cost, within private homes or other community-based settings (National Academy on an Aging Society, 2000; Stone, 2000; Tennstedt, 1999). If informal supports such as these were not available, the long-term care costs of older adults would more than double (Arno, Levine, & Memmott, 1999). The cost of elder care is projected to grow from 38% of total health care costs to nearly 75% when the population of adults over age 65 doubles, between 2000 and 2030 (Evashwick, 2001; Feinberg, 2001).

These dramatic expenditures result in part from the following factors: the increase in the number of people age 85 and older, who have the highest risk of multiple health problems, physical frailty and cognitive impairment; the extended longevity of people experiencing significant disabilities earlier in life; and the 49% increase in the age 65+ cohort by 2010 (U.S. Administration on Aging, 2000; U.S. Census Bureau, 1999). Although informal care to elders is not a new phenomenon, it now is typically more intensive and technologically demanding, of longer duration, and is provided for multiple family members (Bengston, 2001). Current state and federal pressure to reduce health care costs–including hospital downsizing and cuts to managed care and Medicaid–place even greater demands on informal supports. Given these national trends, the identification of vulnerable caregivers and factors that support or hinder their ability to provide high-quality care are critical practice, research, and policy issues.

As a result of their history of disadvantage, marginalization, and invisibility, LGBT caregivers and care receivers may encounter distinct obstacles in securing support, including discrimination in health care and long-term care settings, limited access to services, and the lack of legal protection for their partners and other loved ones. Such obstacles may be encountered if the caregiver and/or care receiver are members of the LGBT community. These unique and challenging circumstances suggest that caregivers and care receivers in LGBT communities may be at especially high risk for deleterious health and caregiving outcomes.

In this introduction we will examine what is currently known about caregiving in LGBT communities, including the prevalence of caregiving responsibilities and the unique structural issues that have been identified as differentiating LGBT caregiving from other types of informal care. Lastly, we will outline the topics that are included in this special edition to advance our understanding of caregiving within historically disadvantaged communities and to create a blueprint for future development in services, research and policies to better meet the growing needs of caregivers and those receiving care.

PREVALENCE AND CAREGIVING PROVIDED

Although an accurate assessment is difficult given the ambiguities of defining sexual orientation as well as the reluctance to self-identify, estimates of the proportion of the population who are lesbian, gay or bisexual range from as low as 2% to as high as 18-20% (Sell, Wells, & Wypij, 1995; Tanfer, 1993; Cahill et al., 2000). Michael, Gagnon, Lauman and Kolata (1994) found, in one of the largest representative data sets available, that 5% of males and 4% of females had engaged in same-sex sexual behavior since the age of 18. Based on a reinterpretation of the Kinsey findings and related research, it is generally estimated that 2.4%-10% of the population is lesbian, gay or bisexual (Cahill et al., 2000).

An analysis of the 2000 U.S. Census data found that 594,391 households self-identified as same-sex unmarried partners, representing nearly 1.2 million gay men and lesbian adults (Bradford, Barrett, & Honnold, 2002). The older lesbian and gay male population is projected to grow from approximately two to over six million by the year 2030 because of the significant overall increase in the older population (Berger, 1996; Cahill, South & Spade, 2000). There are currently no population estimates for transgender individuals, although in 1996 it was reported that more than 25,000 persons had obtained sex reassignment surgery and more than 60,000 planned to do so (Goldberg, 1996).

LGBT individuals are tremendously diverse with respect to sexual orientation, gender identity, age, ethnicity and race, culture, geographic location, education, income, family relationships, health and physical abilities; and these important differences must be recognized in any discussion of caregiving. For many LGBT persons, their families encompass both family of origin and family of choice, including partners, children, grandchildren, parents, grandparents, and other biological relatives, as well as intimate friends and other extended family members. Caregiving in LGBT communities may occur through a variety of relationships: they may be caring for or receiving care from partners, friends, parents, children, and grandparents, as well as neighbors and others.

LGBT individuals, like other caregivers, tend to assist their loved ones with a wide spectrum of illnesses and disabilities and to provide a range of caregiving assistance, including instrumental activities inside and outside the home (e.g., transportation, meal preparation, and housework), personal care (e.g., bathing, feeding, and dressing), emotional support, financial assistance, and mediating with formal services. Contrary to the myth that LGBT persons do not have families, the first national study on lesbian and gay caregiving across the lifespan found that they have extensive caregiving responsibilities; for example, 32% of the gay men and lesbians were providing some type of informal care, ranging from the care of children to the care of adults with serious illness or disability (Fredriksen, 1999). Among the 27% providing adult care, 23% were assisting someone age 18-64 and 8% were assisting someone 65 or older. Among the caregivers providing care for ill and disabled adults, the majority of those they cared for were friends (61%), followed by parents (16%), partners (13%), and other biological family members (10%).

In another early study at a large worksite setting, 13% of the sample that were taking care of a disabled or sick partner or spouse were in a same-sex relationship (Fredriksen, 1996). More recently among lesbians and gay men 50 and older in New York, 8% reported a current need for assistance while 19% had needed care in the past (Cantor, Brennan & Shippy, 2004). Among lesbian, gay male and bisexual adults 50 and older, 45% were currently providing care to a partner, friend or biological family member, usually a parent (Cahill, Ellen, & Tobias, 2002). In a recent study of 32 pairs of LGBT care recipients age 50 and older and their caregivers one-half were partners, 44% were friends, 3% were members of their biological family (most often siblings) and 3% were neighbors and others (Fredriksen-Goldsen & Muraco, 2006).

RISK FACTORS

Historical Context

Some studies suggest that aging experiences are qualitatively different as a result of the double stigma experienced from the intersection of age and sexual orientation (Connidis, 2001; Gabbay & Wahler, 2002; Wojciechowski, 1998). The current cohort of older LGBT individuals has lived through historical periods marked by active hostility toward them. The severe stigmatization as well as the historical context and negative attitudes toward LGBT caregivers and care receivers likely influence caregiving experiences and outcomes, affecting not only the attitudes of family members, friends, and helping professionals, but also self-disclosure and help-seeking behaviors among LGBT adults.

Self-Disclosure

De Monteflores and Schultz (1978) define coming out as "the developmental process through which gay people recognize their sexual preferences and choose to integrate this knowledge into their lives" (p. 59). Coming out is a normative life-long developmental process that requires LGBT persons to remake a stigmatized identity into a positive one. Research to date suggests a positive correlation between one's psychological health and being honest and open about one's sexual orientation (Rand, Graham, & Rawlings, 1982; Weinberg & Williams, 1974), except in those cases involving highly vulnerable populations, such as very frail and ailing individuals, for whom "coming out" is perceived as especially threatening (Cole, Kemeny, & Taylor, 1997).

Unlike some other minority groups, LGBT persons are not readily identifiable; thus, as caregivers and care receivers, they may monitor and manage the issue of disclosure of their sexual orientation or gender identity and the nature of their primary relationships. Insufficient disclosure can result in the restriction of one's support system, while readily disclosing can expose an individual to hostility from the outside world (Gonsiorek, 1995). Yet, the extent of self-disclosure determines the nature and depth of one's support system, and a high degree of social support available to a caregiver has repeatedly been found to be associated with more positive caregiving outcomes (Magana, 1999). Furthermore, caregiving itself often results in the restriction of personal and social opportunities (Callery, 2000; Clipp, Adinolfi, Forrest, & Bennett, 1995; Turner, Catania, & Gagnon, 1994), which compounds any restriction resulting from lack of disclosure of one's identity or personal relationships to family, friends or service providers.

Kinship Relations

In the general caregiving literature, kinship ties have been found to be related to the extent and pattern of care received. Among those in the general population, more than 50% of older adults outside institutional settings and needing assistance rely primarily on family to help with daily activities–typically their adult children (42%), followed by their spouses (25%) (National Academy on an Aging Society, 2000). In general, biological family members tend to be a primary source of support for caregivers. However, LGBT caregivers may receive less support than they need from their own or the care recipient's family of origin. On the one hand, they may be expected to provide unrealistic levels of caregiving assistance within their families of origin, due to an assumption that their partners and close friends are of less importance and do not constitute family.

Contrary to existing stereotypes, most gay men and lesbians caring for a disabled adult do receive some support from their biological families: only 7% reported no support whatsoever from biological family members, while 68% received at least *some* support and 25% reported that their entire family was supportive of them (Fredriksen, 1999). Although perhaps supportive, a few studies suggest that biological family members may not be as actively involved in helping them meet their caregiving responsibilities when they are providing assistance to disabled partners, friends, or others in their extended support network (Aronson, 1998; Hash, 2001; Hash & Cramer, 2003). Among lesbians and gay men 50 and older, the vast majority report that they would go to their partners first for assistance; among those without partners, most would seek assistance from their friends (Cahill et al., 2002).

Support Services

In the general caregiving literature, it has been found that caregivers experiencing diminished access to formal support systems face significantly more physical, psychological, emotional, social, and financial risks (George & Gwyther, 1986). LGBT caregivers and care recipients have been found to be less likely to benefit from formal services, both because of providers' insensitivity and prejudice as well as their own reluctance to utilize formal services. Unfortunately, many LGBT caregivers and care receivers are reluctant to openly acknowledge their sexual orientation or gender identity and their primary relationships in formal care settings because of fear of prejudice among service providers.

Prejudice expressed by professionals or embedded in services can be subtle or blatant (Coon, 2003). Service providers may fail to acknowledge or may openly disregard significant relationships within LGBT families. Others may discredit the role of these caregivers by, for example, more readily providing biological family members with information. Furthermore, biases may be so deeply embedded into the delivery of services that they limit or deny access such as not allowing visitation rights in hospital settings.

For reasons such as these, LGBT caregivers and care recipients tend to not seek out supplementary support or formal services, even when it is understood that there is a need for specialized care (Tully, 1989). Those that conceal their sexual orientation or gender identity may be the most isolated and in need of assistance, yet the least likely to use formal support services. It is generally assumed that patients receive higher quality and more thorough care when they are able to be honest and open with their health care and social service providers (Lambda Legal, 2003; Nystrom, 1997; Robertson, 2003). It is important to note that support services developed within LGBT communities may lack sensitivity to aging issues and tend to be most utilized by individuals who openly self-identify.

Discrimination and Lack of Legal Protection

Discrimination and prejudice intensify risk factors for LGBT caregivers and recipients. For example, as many as 94% of lesbians and gay men report experiencing some type of harassment or discrimination due to their sexual orientation (National Gay and Lesbian Task Force, 1990). The majority of gay men and lesbians providing care to an ill or disabled adult also report experiencing harassment related to their sexual orientation, including verbal (93%), emotional (46%), physical (14%), and sexual (8%) (Fredriksen, 1999).

Lack of support and discrimination at the workplace may place LGBT individuals at higher risk for negative caregiving outcomes. Unsupportive workplaces will likely fail to recognize the legitimacy of their relationships and caregiving responsibilities, which may increase caregiving stress by denying them the day-to-day emotional support and access to workplace benefits that are accorded to other families in similar situations.

Many federal and state laws and policies that provide family-based benefits are inherently biased against LGBT caregivers and care recipients. The range of institutional inequities includes: denying same-sex partners health care benefits and family leave; not providing for equivalent Medicaid spend-downs, social security benefits or bereavement leave; and exclusionary requirements in some managed care and insurance policies. If extensive legal planning is not completed in advance, LGBT caregivers' and care recipients' wishes and decisions may not be honored, especially if they conflict with the desires of biological family members. Yet, in one recent study it was found that the majority of LGBT care recipients and their caregivers do not have sufficient legal protections; for example, among LGBT care recipients 60% do not have a will despite the fact that many are living with serious disabling health conditions (Fredriksen-Goldsen & Muraco, 2006). Fifty-three percent of their caregivers also had not executed a will. In terms of a durable power of attorney for health care, 50% of the LGBT care recipients and 50% of their caregivers did not have one.

Caregiving Outcomes

The majority of general caregiving studies suggest that informal care for a relative with disabilities results in negative consequences for caregivers and their families (Owens, 2001; Polen & Green, 2001). In the general caregiving research, caregiving strain is repeatedly associated with decreased physical and psychological health among caregivers, including increased levels of caregiver burden (Braithwaite, 2000), role strain, fatigue (Polen & Green, 2001), anxiety (Cochrane, Goering, & Rogers, 1997; Polen & Green, 2001), depression (Berg-Weger, Rubio, & Tebb, 2000; Han & Haley, 1999) and poor health outcomes over time (Beach, Schulz, Yee, & Jackson, 2000). In terms of mortality, spousal caregivers who report caregiving strain are 63 percent more likely to die within four years when compared to matched controls (Schultz & Beach, 1999).

Little is known about the physical and psychological health of LGBT caregivers and care receivers. Hash (2001) reported increased risk for physical and psychological strain, poor nutrition, and financial problems among gay male and lesbian caregivers. In addition, a few community-based surveys have documented relatively high levels of physical, financial, and emotional strain among LGBT caregivers (Fredriksen, 1999; Hoctel, 2002; Shippy, Cantor, & Brennan, 2001). Employed caregivers assisting ill and disabled same-sex partners, as compared to opposite-sex partners, provide significantly more hours of care and higher levels of assistance as well as higher levels of role strain and increased likelihood of job termination as a result of their care responsibilities (Fredriksen, 1996). In a recent LGBT caregiving study, care recipients, as compared to their caregivers, were found to have significantly higher levels of depression and strain combined with poor health (Fredriksen-Goldsen & Muraco, 2006); although care recipients are most often left out of caregiving studies, 68% of the care recipients had clinical levels of depression as did 43% of their caregivers.

At the same time, research demonstrates a high level of resilience among LGBT elders, likely due to the capacities they have developed through surmounting obstacles as members of a disadvantaged and disenfranchised group (Berger, 1996; Clunis, Fredriksen-Goldsen, Freeman, & Nystrom, 2005). Their skills at both adaptation and role flexibility need to be further explored as they may help them in meeting caregiving demands.

MOVING FORWARD

Caregiving is changing dramatically as a result of the growing elder population, the increasing diversity of families, and on-going shifts in health and long-term care services. The research described in this collection illustrates the significance of caregiving and care receiving within LGBT communities and highlights the importance to further understand the diversity of caregiving experiences, the impact of these responsibilities and the resulting needs of caregivers and their loved ones within marginalized communities.

In this volume, Grossman, D'Augelli, and Dragowski explore the prevalence of caregiving and care receiving among lesbian, gay, and bisexual (LGB) older adults, and their willingness to offer care in the future. Next, Shippy examines not only the burdens of caregiving, but also the impact of stigma and discrimination and social support on both family of origin and family of choice caregivers. Based on a framework of caregiving resilience, Fredriksen-Goldsen considers the extent of variations in HIV/AIDS caregiving outcomes and what risk and protective factors impact caregiver distress and well-being.

Illustrating the significance of the cultural context, Evans-Campbell and her colleagues explore contemporary experiences as well as the historical roles of caregiving among Native American Indian two-spirit people and the implications of these roles within Native communities.

Research on the lives and concerns of transgender elders is presented by Williams and Freeman; their analysis illuminates important issues that must be considered if effective and respectful interventions are to be developed to support transgender elders and their caregivers across the life course.

Providing an overview of intervention issues and strategies designed to assist caregivers, Coon describes a community-based intervention specifically developed to assist LGBT caregivers. Lastly, Fredriksen-Goldsen and Hooyman explore ways to increase both theoretical and methodological rigor in future research, and outline a blueprint for service and policy development to sustain caregivers, care receivers and their loved ones in marginalized communities.

As we move forward in caregiving research, services and policies, this volume provides a unique opportunity to explore the realities and possibilities for caregiving across diverse communities.

REFERENCES

Arno, P. S., Levine, C., & Memmott, M. M. (1999). The economic value of informal caregiving. *Health Affairs, 18,* 182-188.

Aronson, J. (1998). Lesbians giving and receiving care: Stretching conceptualizations of caring and community. *Women's Studies International Forum, 21*(5), 505-519.

Badgett, M. V. L. (1998). *Income inflation: The myth of affluence among gay, lesbian, and bisexual Americans.* New York: The Policy Institute of the National Gay & Lesbian Task Force.

Beach, S., Schulz, R., Yee, J., & Jackson, S. (2000). Negative and positive health effects of caring for a disabled spouse: Longitudinal findings from the Caregiver Health Effects Study. *Psychology and Aging, 15*(2), 259-271.

Bengston, V. L. (2001). Beyond the nuclear family: The increasing importance of multigenerational bonds. *Journal of Marriage and the Family, 63,* 1-16.

Berger, R. M. (1996). *Gay and gray: The older homosexual man (2nd. ed.).* Binghamton, NY: The Haworth Press.

Berg-Weger, M., Rubio, D. M., & Tebb, S. S. (2000). Depression as a mediator: Viewing caregiver well-being and strain in a different light. *Families in Society: The Journal of Contemporary Human Services, 81*(2), 162-173.

Bradford, J., Barrett, K., & Honnold, J. A. (2002). *The 2000 census and same-sex households: A user's guide.* New York: The Policy Institute of the National Gay & Lesbian Task Force, the Survey and Evaluation Research Laboratory, and the Fenway Institute.

Braithwaite, V. (2000). Making choices through caregiving appraisals. *The Gerontologist, 40,* 706-717.

Brody, E. (1985). Parent care as a normative family stress. *Gerontologist, 25,* 19-29.

Brotman, S., Ryan, B., & Cormier, R. (2003). The health and social service needs of gay and lesbian elders and their families in Canada. *The Gerontologist, 43*(2), 192.

Cahill, S., Ellen, M., & Tobias, S. (2002). *Family policy: Issues affecting gay, lesbian, bisexual, and transgender families.* New York: The Policy Institute of the National Gay & Lesbian Task Force.

Cahill, S., South, K., & Spade, J. (2000). *Outing age: Public policy issues affecting gay, lesbian, bisexual, and transgender elders.* (Policy Report). New York: The Policy Institute of the National Gay & Lesbian Task Force.

Callery, K. E. (2000). The role of stigma and psycho-social factors on perceived caregiver burden in HIV/AIDS gay male caregivers. *Dissertation Abstracts International: Section B: The Sciences and Engineering, 61*(5-B), 2469.

Cantor, M. H., Brennan, M., & Shippy, R. A. (2004). *Caregiving among older lesbian, gay, bisexual and transgender New Yorkers.* (Policy Report). New York: The Policy Institute of the National Gay and Lesbian Task Force.

Clipp, E. C., Adinolfi, A. J., Forrest, L., & Bennett, C. L. (1995). Informal caregivers of persons with AIDS. *Journal of Palliative Care, 11*(2), 10-18.

Clunis, M., Fredriksen-Goldsen, K. I., Freeman, P., & Nystrom, N. (2005). *Looking back, looking forward: The lives of lesbian elders.* Binghamton, NY: The Haworth Press.

Cochrane, J. J., Goering, P. N., & Rogers, J. M. (1997). The mental health of informal caregivers in Ontario: An epidemiological survey. *American Journal of Public Health, 87,* 2002-2007.

Cole, S. W., Kemeny, M. E., & Taylor, S. E. (1997). Social identity and physical health: Accelerated HIV progression in rejection-sensitive gay men. *Journal of Personality and Social Psychology, 72*(2), 320-335.

Connidis, I. (2001). *Family Ties and Aging.* Thousand Oaks, CA: Sage Publications.

Coon, D. W. (2003). *Lesbian, gay, bisexual, and transgender (LGBT) issues and family caregiving.* San Francisco, CA: Family Caregiver Alliance National Center on Caregiving.

De Monteflores, C., & Schultz, S. (1978). Coming out: Similarities and differences for lesbians and gay men. *Journal of Social Issues, 34,* 59-72.

Evashwick, C. J. (2001). *The continuum of long-term care: An integrated systems approach.* Albany, NY: Delmar Learning.

Feinberg, L. F. (2001). *Systems development for family caregiver support services.* San Francisco, CA: Family Caregiver Alliance.

Fredriksen, K. I. (1996, July). *Lesbian and gay caregiving.* Paper presented at the 18th Annual National Lesbian and Gay Health Conference, Seattle, WA.

Fredriksen, K. I. (1999). Family caregiving responsibilities among lesbians and gay men. *Social Work, 44*(2), 142-155.

Fredriksen-Goldsen, K. I. (2003). *Resiliency and AIDS caregiving: Predictors of well-being and distress.* Paper presented at the 56th Annual Scientific Meeting of the Gerontological Society of America, San Diego, CA, November, 2003.

Fredriksen-Goldsen, K. I., Muraco, A. Caregiving in the margins: The impact of the caring relationship. Paper presented at the 59th Annual Scientific Meeting of the Gerontological Society of America, Dallas, Texas, November, 2006.

Gabbay, S. G., & Wahler, J. J. (2002). Lesbian aging: Review of a growing literature. *Journal of Gay & Lesbian Social Services, 14*(3), 1-21.

Garnets, L., Hancock, K., Cochran, S., Goodchilds, J., & Peplau, L. (1991). Issues in psychotherapy with lesbians and gay men: A survey of psychologists. *American Psychologist, 46,* 964-972.

George, L. K., & Gwyther, L. P. (1986). Caregiver well-being: A multidimensional examination of family caregivers of demented adults. *Gerontologist, 26*(3), 253-259.

Goldberg, C. (1996, September 8). He and she, they fight for respect. *New York Times,* 10.

Gonsiorek, J. C. (1995). Gay male identities: Concepts and issues. In A. R. D' Augelli & C. J. Patterson (Eds.), *Lesbian, gay, and bisexual identities over the lifespan: Psychological perspectives* (pp. 24-47). New York: Oxford University Press.

Han, B., & Haley, W. E. (1999). Family caregiving for patients with stroke: Review and analysis. *Stroke, 30,* 1478-1485.

Hancock, K. A. (2000). Lesbian, gay, and bisexual lives: Basic issues in psychotherapy training and practice. In B. Green & G. L. Croom (Eds.), *Education, research, and practice in lesbian, gay, bisexual, and transgendered psychology* (pp. 91-130). Thousand Oaks, CA: Sage Publications.

Hash, K. M. (2001). Preliminary study of caregiving and post-caregiving experiences of older gay men and lesbians. *Journal of Gay & Lesbian Social Services, 13*(4), 87-94.

Hash, K. M., & Cramer, E. P. (2003). Empowering gay and lesbian caregivers and uncovering their unique experiences through the use of qualitative methods. *Journal of Gay & Lesbian Social Services, 15*(1/2), 47-63.

Hoctel, P. D. (2002, January-February). Community assessments show service gaps for LGBT elders. *Aging Today, 23*(1), 5-6.

Kauth, M. R., Hartwig, M. J., & Kalichman, S. C. (2000). Health behavior relevant to psychotherapy with lesbian, gay, and bisexual clients. In R. Perez, K. A. DeBord, and K. J. Bieschke (Eds.), *Handbook of counseling and psychotherapy with lesbian, gay, and bisexual clients* (pp. 435-446). Washington, DC: American Psychological Association.

Lambda Legal. (2003). *Brooklyn Housing v. Lynch: New case!* Washington, DC: Author.

Magana, S. M. (1999). Puerto Rican families caring for an adult with mental retardation: Role of famialism. *American Journal on Mental Retardation, 104*(5), 466.

Michael, M. T., Gagnon, E. O., Laumann, J. H., & Kolata, G. B. (1995). *Sex in America: A Definitive Survey.* New York: Warner Books

National Academy on an Aging Society. (2000). Helping the elderly with activity limitations. Paper presented at Caregiving #7, Washington, D.C.

National Gay & Lesbian Task Force. (1990). *Anti-gay violence, victimization and defamation in 1989.* Washington, DC: Author.

Nystrom, N. M. (1997). Oppression by mental health providers: A report by gay men and lesbians about their treatment. *Dissertation Abstracts International. 58*(6-A), 2394.

Owens, S. D. (2001). African American female elder caregivers: An analysis of the psychosocial correlates of their stress level, alcohol use and psychological well-being. *Dissertation Abstracts International: Humanities and Social Sciences, 62*(1), 332A-333A.

Phillips, J., & Fischer, A. (1998). Graduate students' training experiences with lesbian, gay, and bisexual issues. *Counseling Psychologist, 26,* 712-734.

Polen, M. R., & Green, C.A. (2001). Caregiving, alcohol use and mental health symptoms among HMO members. *Journal of Community Health, 26*(4), 285-301.

Rand, C., Graham, D. L. R., & Rawlings, E. I. (1982). Psychological health and factors the court seeks to control in lesbian mother custody trials. *Journal of Homosexuality, 8,* 27-39.

Robertson, P. A. (2003). Offering high-quality ob/gyn care to lesbian patients. *Contemporary Ob/Gyn, September,* 49-56.

Schulz, R. & Beach, S. (1999). Caregiving as a risk factor for mortality: The Caregiver Health Effects Study. *Journal of the American Medical Association, 282*(23), 2215-2219.

Sell, R. L., Wells, J. A., & Wypij, D. (1995). The prevalence of homosexual behavior and attraction in the United States, the United Kingdom, and France: Results of a national population-based sample. *Archives of Sexual Behavior, 24,* 235-248.

Shippy, R. A., Cantor, M. H., & Brennan, M. (2001, November). *Patterns of Support for Lesbians and Gay Men as They Age.* In M. H. Cantor (Chair), *Social Support Networks.* Symposium held at the 54th Annual Scientific Meeting of the Gerontological Society of America, Chicago, IL.

Stone, R. I. (2000). *Long-term care for the elderly with disabilities: Current policy, emerging trends, and implications for the twenty-first century.* New York,: Milbank Memorial Fund.

Tanfer, K. (1993). National survey of men: Design and execution. *Family Planning Perspectives, 25,* 83-86.

Tennstedt, S. (1999). *Family Caregivers In An Aging Society.* U.S. Administration on Aging Symposium on Longevity in the New American Century: Baltimore, MD.

Tully, C. T. (1989). What do midlife lesbians view as important? *Journal of Gay & Lesbian Psychotherapy, 1*(1), 87-103.

Turner, H. A., Catania, J. A., & Gagnon, J. (1994). The prevalence of informal caregiving to persons with AIDS in the United States: Caregiver characteristics and their implications. *Social Science and Medicine, 38*(11), 1543-1552.

U.S. Administration on Aging. (2000). *Profile of older Americans.* Washington, DC: Author.

U.S. Census Bureau. (1999). *Population Projections of the United States: Current Population Reports* (P60, N198). Washington, DC: U.S. Department of Commerce.

Weinberg, M. S., & Williams, C. S. (1974). *Male homosexuals: Their problems and adaptations.* New York: Oxford University Press.

Wenzel, H. V. (2002). *Fact sheet: Legal issues for LGBT caregivers* (Fact Sheet). San Francisco, CA: Family Caregiver Alliance.

Winegarten, B., Cassie, N., Markowski, K., Kozlowski, J., & Yoder, J. (1994). *Aversive heterosexism: Exploring unconscious bias toward lesbian psychotherapy clients.* Paper presented at the 102nd Annual Convention of the American Psychological Association, Los Angeles, CA.

Wojciechowski, C. (1998). Issues in caring for older lesbians. *Journal of Gerontological Nursing [NLM-MEDLINE], 24*(7), 28-34.

doi:10.1300/J041v18n03_01

Caregiving and Care Receiving Among Older Lesbian, Gay, and Bisexual Adults

Arnold H. Grossman
Anthony R. D'Augelli
Eliza A. Dragowski

SUMMARY. A survey research design was used to examine caregiving, care receiving, and the willingness to provide caregiving among lesbian, gay, and bisexual (LGB) older adults recruited from community groups. More than one-third reported receiving care from people other than healthcare providers in the last five years; more than two thirds provided care to other LGB adults. Those who had given care were more likely than non-caregivers to give care in the future. The gender and sexual orientation

Arnold H. Grossman, PhD, is Professor, Department of Applied Psychology, New York University, 239 Greene Street, Suite 400, New York, NY 10003 (E-mail: arnold. grossman@nyu.edu).

Anthony R. D'Augelli, PhD, is Professor, Department of Human Development and Family Studies, The Pennsylvania State University, 105Q White Building, University Park, PA 16802 (E-mail: ard@psu.edu).

Eliza A. Dragowski, PhD, is Research Assistant, Department of Applied Psychology, New York University, 239 Greene Street, Suite 400, New York, NY 10003 (E-mail: ead218@nyu.edu).

The authors acknowledge the staff and volunteers of the agencies and groups who co-operated in recruiting participants. Timothy O'Connell is thanked for assistance with the research design, and planning and organization skills that helped the project begin. The authors also thank the study participants. This research was supported by the Research Challenge Fund of New York University's Steinhardt School of Education.

[Haworth co-indexing entry note]: "Caregiving and Care Receiving Among Older Lesbian, Gay, and Bisexual Adults." Grossman, Arnold H., Anthony R. D'Augelli, and Eliza A. Dragowski. Co-published simultaneously in *Journal of Gay & Lesbian Social Services* (The Haworth Press, Inc.) Vol. 18, No. 3/4, 2007, pp. 15-38; and: *Caregiving with Pride* (ed: Karen I. Fredriksen-Goldsen) The Haworth Press, Inc., 2007, pp. 15-38. Single or multiple copies of this article are available for a fee from The Haworth Document Delivery Service [1-800-HAWORTH, 9:00 a.m. - 5:00 p.m. (EST). E-mail address: docdelivery@haworthpress.com].

Available online at http://jglss.haworthpress.com
doi:10.1300/J041v18n03_02

of recipients of future help affected participants' willingness to provide care, as did their education level and style of coping. Participants willing to provide care to older LGB adults perceived such experiences to be less burdensome and more personally rewarding than those who were unwilling to provide care. doi:10.1300/J041v18n03_02 *[Article copies available for a fee from The Haworth Document Delivery Service: 1-800-HAWORTH. E-mail address: <docdelivery@haworthpress.com> Website: <http://www. HaworthPress.com> © 2007 by The Haworth Press, Inc. All rights reserved.]*

KEYWORDS. Homosexuality, sexual orientation, caregiving, care receiving, aging, older adults

INTRODUCTION

Gerontological literature indicates that family members are the primary source of care for the elderly (Dwyer & Coward, 1992; Harris & Bichler, 1997). Despite advances in institutional long-term care of physically ill and functionally impaired elderly adults, a shift to community-based services and informal family support systems continues. It is estimated that 80% of all caregiving for older people in the United States is done informally by the family (Matthews & Rosner, 1988). However, having family members (i.e., biological kin) serve as primary care providers may not be an option for many older lesbian, gay, and bisexual (LGB) adults because of their estranged relationships with them. These LGB adults moved through adulthood during a period in which their same-sex attractions were considered symptoms of mental disorder, their behavior and lifestyles were judged immoral by virtually all religions, and their consensual sexual activities were illegal (Rubenstein, 1996).[1] To avoid rejection and the stigma associated with their sexual orientation, some older LGB people moved away from their biological families and communities of origin to cities with more tolerance, thereby separating themselves from potential family caregivers (Harris, 1981); in addition, they continued to conceal their sexual orientation from family members (Brotman, Ryan, & Cormier, 2003; Thomas, 1996). Many of these older adults are now concerned about who will provide care if they become physically or mentally impaired. This concern is intensified for those living alone and those with few LGB friends or connections to a LGB community (Porter, Russell, & Sullivan, 2004).

Grossman, D'Augelli and Hershberger (2000) found that one-third of a sample of 416 LGB adults over 60 years of age had never told their parents, siblings, or relatives about their sexual orientation. Older LGB adults who have told family members and found them to be unaccepting would have fewer kin to rely on for caregiving than comparable older heterosexual adults. Neither the caregiving needs of older LGB adults nor the caregiving practices of older LGB people have been examined in the gerontological literature (Cahill, South, & Spade, 2000).

Fredriksen (1999), examining caregiving activities of 1,466 people directed toward their families (their own parents or children in same-sex families), found that many LG adults were providing care for others. One-third of the LG people in her study were engaged in caregiving; of those assisting adults with illnesses or disabilities, 61% were caring for friends. Gay men were found to be more likely to be caring for working-age adults, many of whom were dealing with HIV-related health problems, whereas lesbians more often cared for children and people aged 65 or older. However, Fredriksen (1999) did not study the sexual orientation of the older adults receiving care.

Traditionally, most caregiving has been done by women, mainly wives and daughters; however, husbands and sons are increasingly giving care (Harris & Bichler, 1997). Little empirical evidence of this phenomenon is available about those LGB people providing care or willing to provide care.

An additional problem is that older LGB adults may be reluctant to turn for help to social service agencies. A Canadian qualitative study (Brotman et al., 2003), using 32 LG seniors and their families, found that many elderly gay men and lesbians mistrusted health and social service agencies, and were reluctant to seek health care. Using a sample of 71 LGB adults aged 50 to 80, Jacobs, Rasmussen and Hohman (1999) found that many older LGB adults evaluated social service agencies specifically dedicated to lesbian and gay clients more positively than other services.

Concerns about adequate caregiving for LGB adults may seem paradoxical as this group is often considered to have strong social support networks (Grossman et al., 2000). Quam and Whitford (1992), studying adaptation and age-related expectations of 80 lesbian and gay adults over 50, found that more than half participated in a lesbian or gay social group, whereas only 9% participated in local senior centers. Dorfman and her colleagues (1995), using a sample of 108 lesbian, gay, and heterosexual older adults aged 60 to 93, found lesbians and gay men received significantly more support from friends, while heterosexual elderly derived more support from biological family members. In a study of 160 lesbians and gay men aged 45 to 90, Beeler, Rawls, Herdt, and Cohler (1999) found that more than two-thirds

(68%) had a "family of choice," non-biologically related friends with whom they socialized. Grossman et al. (2000) found that older LGB adults felt more satisfied with support received from people in their networks who knew their sexual orientation.

If older LGB individuals report such social support, why do some feel they cannot count on people in these networks to provide caregiving? Several hypotheses can be forwarded. Receiving social support from friends is quite different than receiving care related to a physical or mental health problem. It is unusual for non-kin to be engaged in caregiving that involves personal care, especially for chronic conditions, unless the caregiver and care recipients are psychologically intimate, such as domestic or dating partners. On the other hand, it is likely that LGB people, over the course of their lives, have received some care from other LGB people who are non-kin (Weston, 1991). This would suggest that perceived reciprocity of caregiving is an issue, with LGB adults being willing to give care to LGB people to the degree that they have received care in the past. It may also be that the specific nature of past caregiving experiences influences future willingness to care for others. For example, someone who has cared for several friends with HIV/AIDS might feel less willing to volunteer more help of this nature due to physical and psychological burdens associated with this care (Turner, Pearlin, & Mullan, 1998). Also, some LGB people may be willing to provide care for certain kinds of LGB people. Based on Grossman et al.'s (2000) findings, one would expect that gay men would be more willing to care for other gay men, and lesbians for lesbians. This is a function of the differential proportions of gay men and lesbians in men's and women's social networks, as well as greater closeness and empathy with people of the same sex.

Although correlates of caregiving have been studied extensively by gerontologists, little research has focused on caregiving for older LGB adults, especially the characteristics of LGB people willing to serve as caregivers for older LGB adults. This issue is important as health and mental health problems specific to this population are identified (Grossman, D'Augelli, & O'Connell, 2001) and as the HIV epidemic continues among older adults (Goodkin et al., 2003). Although Turner et al. (1998), in their study of caregivers of people with AIDS, did not obtain information about the sexual orientation of the adults receiving care, they did about the helpers; many of the "nonfamily" member caregivers studied were gay men who were presumably caring for their partners or for gay friends. The only available study of older gay and lesbian adults' caregiving for other LG people is a qualitative study of 19 middle-aged and older gay men and lesbians caring for chronically ill same-sex partners (Hash, 2001). Caregivers reported experiencing physical and emotional strains; however, they also valued the caregiving opportunities as ways to show their strengths and commitment. Both positive and negative effects of caregiving have been found among caregiving people with AIDS (Turner et al., 1998).

Research is needed on factors related to willingness of LGB adults to provide care to older LGB adults. Useful information includes previous caregiving experiences, burdens, and rewards, as well as information about such characteristics as the sex and sexual orientations of those predisposed to providing care. It is also important to learn if the gender role-based caregiving patterns found among heterosexual women and men are also occurring in the LGB community.

Caring for an elderly person who is physically ill or is impaired can be a demanding task, with negative and positive psychological consequences for the caregiver. Accordingly, most studies examining the impact of caregiving for older adults have used a stress and coping model (Goodkin et al., 2003; Pearlin, Mullan, Semple, & Skaff, 1990). The model suggests that different levels of stressors and resources influence caregiver outcomes (Goode, Haley, Roth, & Ford, 1998; Harris & Bichler, 1997; Zarit, Reever, & Bach-Peterson, 1980). As implied by the buffering hypothesis, those individuals who experience a significant amount of stress as a result of caregiving need resources to buffer or protect them from the detrimental effects of that stress (Cohen & Wills, 1985). One common caregiver outcome linked to stress is caregiver burden, which has both objective and subjective aspects. Objective burden concerns disruption or change in caregivers' lives, whereas subjective burden concerns attitudes or emotional reactions to the caregiving experience (Montgomery, Gonyea, & Hooyman, 1985; Vitaliano, Young, & Russo, 1991). Feeling burdened is an important consequence of caregiving, and the expectation of future caregiving burden is likely to influence one's willingness to provide help. Other related factors commonly associated with caregiving to others are perceived personal stress, the need for more social support from others, problems of one's own health and well-being, and the need to withdraw from one's social networks (Turner et al., 1998). Following these lines of thinking, we adopted the stress and coping model as the conceptual framework for this study.

Another aspect of the stress and coping model is the concept of proactive coping. As indicated by Aspinwall and Taylor (1997), proactive coping involves mobilizing resources and preparing strategies to deal with the stress before its onset. Such coping may either prevent the stressor, help cope more effectively with the stressor, or improve well-being after the onset of the stressor. Consequently, knowing the nature of and preparing for future caregiving roles may be useful to older LGB adults who may be called on to be caregivers (Pinquart & Sorenson, 2002). Also, it is important that we learn the characteristics of LGB people willing to serve as caregivers for older LGB adults not only so that we can recruit them in helping and provide for the future care needs of older LGB adults, but also to assist them in learning about the potential benefits and challenges they will face. Unfortunately, most individuals in the United States, including LGB adults, do not have sufficient individual resources and unlimited options for care. And whereas general medical care is covered by Medicare, medical home health care is limited in the amount of time and the types of circumstances for which it is available. Therefore, services can only be accessed by those who have sufficient funds to pay for them or by those who have low enough financial resources to qualify for Medicaid (Sorensen & Pinquart, 2000a).

DESIGN AND METHODS

A survey research design using a self-administered questionnaire was employed. Participants were asked about their caregiving and care-receiving histories, and then queried about their willingness to give care using a standard scale (Wight et al., 1998). Information was also collected about current physical and mental health, loneliness, internalized homophobia, the perceived stresses in one's life, perceived social support, caregiver burden, personal gain from providing care, and coping skills. Demographic information, such as age, gender, ethnicity, education, and income was also obtained. From the perspective of the stress and coping model, we expected that those individuals with lower levels of stress, loneliness and internalized homophobia; better physical and mental health; and more resources, as indicated by higher levels of perceived social support and coping skills, would indicate a greater willingness to provide help with caregiving tasks. We also predicted those individuals with a greater willingness to provide help with caregiving tasks would have lower expectations that it would be burdensome as well as expect more perceived personal gain from helping.

This study used a sample of LGB adults aged 40 to 85 recruited from agencies providing recreational and social services to LGB elders. We focused on factors that gerontological research identified as predictive of future caregiving for older adults, with the ultimate goals of determining characteristics of LGB people willing to serve as caregivers for older LGB adults. The frequencies of care receiving from others and past caregiving were obtained, as well as the relationship between receiving and giving care. We examined the relevance of sex, income, educational level, health, and mental health (Dew et al., 1998; Norris & Kaniasty, 1996) on willingness to provide care. We also studied the expected burden of future caregiving and its personal rewards. Particular factors expected to influence willingness to provide care were internalized homophobia, loneliness, social support, coping skills, and perceived life stress (Grossman et al., 2000; Harris & Bichler, 1997; Montgomery et al., 1995; Norris & Kaniasty, 1996).

Recruitment and Data Collection Procedures

Participants were recruited through five groups and agencies providing social and recreational services to older LGB adults. Three groups were in New York City and two were in Los Angeles, cities that have concentrations of older LGB adults. Contact persons were identified at each site to distribute and collect questionnaires; these were both female and male volunteers. LGB adults had to be 40 years or older,[2] the age at which the agencies begin to provide services for senior citizens. Participants completed questionnaires anonymously and returned them in sealed envelopes to the contact persons. Participants who returned questionnaires provided their names and telephone numbers to be entered into a $100 raffle, used as a recruitment incentive. Data collection took place during 2000 and 2001. The final sample contained 199 LGB adults. A response rate cannot be estimated because only the adults who were willing to complete the questionnaire at the various recreational groups participated in the study, while others who repeatedly attended the groups chose not to participate. Consequently, the findings cannot be generalized to all older LGB adults. Procedures were approved by the IRB's of both universities involved.

Past experiences in giving and receiving care. Twelve caregiving tasks used by Wight, LeBlanc, and Aneshensel (1998) determined caregiving experiences: helping with taking medication, doing housework/cleaning, shopping for food, cooking and preparing food, doing laundry, helping with using transportation, helping with using a telephone, eating, dressing, grooming, bathing and toileting, and getting in and out of bed. Participants were asked how many people they had helped with these tasks in the past five years. Response options were 0, 1, 2 to 5 people, 6 to 10 people, and more than 10 people. They were asked to list the four most recent conditions, illnesses, or diseases of the people they had helped, and how many months were involved in helping people with each problem. Additionally, the participants were asked how often they had provided care for either people with HIV/AIDS or victims of gay-related physical attack (i.e., an attack motivated by homophobia).

As an index of their past experience receiving care from others, they were asked if people *other than health-care providers* had provided them with any of the 12 kinds of help in the last five years. They were asked whether they had never been helped, or helped once, 2 to 5 times, 6 to 10 times, or more than 10 times. They were asked to list up to four "conditions, illnesses, or diseases" for which they received care, and who the helpers were. The "conditions, illnesses, or diseases" for which they gave or received care-giving were categorized by type, e.g., cancer, muscular-skeletal, cardiovascular, gastrointestinal, and chronic diseases associated with aging (such as visual impairments, hearing impairments or deafness, or dementia and other communication impairments).

Willingness to provide care in the future. Using a four-point scale ranging from 4 = *very willing* to 1 = *very unwilling*, participants rated willingness to help with each of the 12 caregiving tasks. So that the ratings would be grounded in a more concrete context, they were asked, *"How willing would you be to help an older LGB person who was home-bound with the following tasks? (For example, think about a situation in which a single older LGB person who has had back surgery needs to recuperate at home for 5-6 weeks in a walk-up apartment. The person received 3 hours of care each morning from a health aide, but needs help from others during the day.)"* The participants' scores for the 12 tasks were averaged as an index of willingness to provide care. Cronbach's alpha was .93. They were also asked which of the following types of people they would be willing to help: gay males, lesbians, bisexuals, and heterosexuals.

Predictors of willingness to provide caregiving to LGB adults. Several other factors were examined for their relationship to future caregiving propensity. Several demographic characteristics were tested, including age, income, and employment status, following Turner et al. (1998). Employment options were employed, retired, or unemployed; and participants' current occupation or their occupation before retirement was used. Participants' health and mental health were assessed with two items used in earlier research on older LGB adults (D'Augelli, Grossman, Hershberger, & O'Connell, 2001): *"How would you describe your physical health at the present time?"* and *"How would you describe your mental and emotional health at the present time?"*–each answered from *Very Poor* to *Excellent* on a five-point scale. Higher scores reflected better physical health and mental health. It was expected that participants with better physical and mental health would be more likely to agree to future caregiving.

Six items from the Revised Homosexuality Attitude Inventory (RHAI; Shidlo, 1994) were used to measure internalized homophobia, or negative feelings about homosexuality. These items were chosen based on item-total correlations with the version of the measure used by D'Augelli et al. (2001). Participants responded to a four-point Likert-type scale, ranging from *strongly agree* to *strongly disagree*. High scores reflected higher internalized homophobia. Cronbach's alpha was .77. Participants with negative views of their own sexual orientation were expected to be less likely to be willing to help other LGB people than participants with more positive attitudes.

Loneliness was measured by three items from the short version of the UCLA Loneliness Scale (Hayes & DiMatteo, 1987). This scale consists of statements (e.g., *"I feel isolated from others"*) rated on a four-point, Likert-type scale (from *strongly agree* to *strongly disagree*). High scores indicated more loneliness. The three items were chosen based on high item-total correlations of the measure from a study of older LGB adults by D'Augelli et al. (2001). Cronbach's alpha was .80. Participants who were less lonely were expected to be more willing to help than those who were lonelier, as loneliness tends to reflect social isolation and an inability to relate to others, and therefore a reluctance to become involved in caregiving.

The Perceived Stress Scale (Cohen, Karmarck, & Mermelstein, 1983) measured perceived level of life stress during the last month. Four items from the scale were chosen based on item-total correlations from D'Augelli et al. (2001). Participants answered questions about how often they felt overwhelmed by recent events, and how effectively they coped with those events (e.g., How often have you felt that you were on top of things?). Items were answered with *never* to *very often*. High scores indicated more life stress. Cronbach's alpha was .71. Participants with higher perceived stress would be expected to be less likely to be willing to provide caregiving than those with less stress, as they would have less psychological resources to bring to the caregiving situation (Turner et al., 1998).

The Perceived Social Support Scale (Norris & Kaniasty, 1996) measured support from others. This nine-question scale contained questions about three types of support: tangible support (e.g., *"If I needed it, I have someone who would go to the doctor with me"*), emotional support (e.g., *"I have someone I feel intimate with"*), and informational support (e.g., *"I have someone who helps me solve problems"*). The statements were assessed on a four-point scale with answers ranging from *definitely true* to *definitely false*. Higher scores reflected more social support. Cronbach's alpha was .93. Social support is important in reducing caregiver stress (e.g., Crystal et al., 2003; Turner et al., 1998), and therefore was expected to be associated with greater willingness to help.

Coping skills were measured using fifteen items from the Coping Inventory for Stressful Situations (CISS; Endler & Parker, 1990), a highly reliable measure of diverse approaches to responding to life stressors. Information was obtained about five kinds of coping: Task-Focused, Emotion-Focused, Avoidance, Distraction, and Social Diversion. Three items from each scale were used, based on item-total correlations from unpublished raw data from D'Augelli and Grossman (2000). A factor analysis of the data in that report of the 15 items revealed two factors, which were used in further calculations. These were: Task-Focused Coping (e.g., *"When I encounter a difficult, stressful, or upsetting situation, I determine a course of action and follow it."*) and Emotion-Focused Coping (e.g., *"When I encounter a difficult, stressful, or upsetting situation, I become very tense"*). Items were rated on a five-point scale ranging from *not at all* to *very much*. A high score indicated a greater tendency to use a particular coping style. Cronbach's alpha was .70 for task-focused coping, and .68 for emotion-focused coping. People who cope in a more task-oriented way tend to show fewer signs of stress, while others who respond emotionally may be less able to manage the stress of caregiving (Hooyman & Lustbader, 1986).

Caregiver burden related to current or past caregiving experience was measured by the Objective Burden Scale and the Subjective Burden Scale (Montgomery et al., 1985). Objective burden was measured by five items on which respondents reported how hypothetical caregiving would change their lives (e.g., *"I'd feel as if I'd put my life on hold"*). Subjective burden was assessed by five items concerning feelings about such caregiving (e.g., *"I'd get nervous and depressed"*). Statements were rated on a four-point scale (from *never* to *all of the time*). Objective and subjective burden scores were significantly correlated, $r(190) = .73$, $p < .001$, so scores were combined into a caregiver burden scale. High scores indicated more expected burden from caregiving. Cronbach's alpha was .87. It was hypothesized that participants who perceived that caregiving would be more burdensome would be less likely to agree to provide caregiving than those perceiving caregiving as less burdensome.

Personal gain from caregiving was assessed with four items recommended by Pearlin et al. (1990). Participants were asked about such consequences of caregiving as becoming aware of their inner strengths and becoming more self-confident. These items were supplemented with three items concerning the respondents' feelings about contributing to the LGB organizations with which they were affiliated, helping LGB people, and building a LGB support group that will be available for them if they needed it later in life. Items were rated on a four-point, Likert-type scale (from *very much* to *not at all*). High scores reflected more personal gain as a result of caring for others. Cronbach's alpha was .87. More willingness to provide care was expected to be associated with perceptions of more personal gain.

Participants

Of the 199 LGB adults, 58% (115) were males and 42% (84) were females, ranging in age from 40 to 85 ($M = 66.02$, $SD = 10.33$). About one quarter (26%, 52) was between 40 and 59 years, while 74% (147) were 60 or older. There were significant differences between those 59 and under and those 60 and older on a number of variables. The younger adults were more likely to have better current physical health, but they had more perceived stress. Also, they were less likely to have a disability. Of the 43% of the participants (86) who had a partner, the younger group reported being in the relationship for fewer years than the older group; however, only 29% (58) of the participants reported living with a lover/partner. Males were significantly older (Male: $M = 69.04$; Female: $M = 62.07$, t (186) = 4.83, $p < .001$). Most (91%, 181) identified as gay or lesbian, and 9% (18) as bisexual. Most (82%, 163) were Caucasian/White, 7% (14) were African-American/Black, 4% (8) were of Hispanic origin, and 7% identified as "other" or of mixed races.

Of the sample, 20% (36) completed high school, 4% (7) a certificate program, 6% (12) an associate degree, 30% (56) a bachelor's degree, 33% (62) a master's degree, 3% (6) a doctorate, and 4% (8) another professional degree. Annual income of participants was as follows: 11% (20) less than $15,000; 26% (46) between $15,000 and $24,999; 18% $25,000 and $34,999; 18% (33) between $35,000 to $49,999; 19% (34) between $50,000 and $74,999; 6% (11) between $75,000 and $100,000; and 2% (4) over $100,000. Most (86%, 171) lived in large cities, 7% (14) in small cities, 6% (12) in the suburbs, and 1% (2) in towns or rural areas.

Data analysis included use of descriptive statistics, *t*-tests, bivariate correlations, and a hierarchical linear regression analysis. Effect sizes using Cohen's d (Cohen, 1988) and his criteria for small ($d = .20$), medium ($d = .50$), and large ($d = .80$) effect sizes are noted in the text.

RESULTS

Past Caregiving and Receiving Care

When asked about care received (e.g., with taking medications, dressing/undressing, eating) from people other than health-care providers in the last five years, more than one-third (38%) of the participants reported such care. Males reported receiving less help than females (31% vs. 46%; χ^2 (1, $N = 197$) = 4.62, $p < .05$). Nine percent reported having been helped once, 13% received care from 2 to 5 times, 7% from 6 to 10 times, and 9% more than 10 times. Participants were divided into two groups: people who had received any care in the last five years and those who had not. Nearly two-thirds (62%) had not received help.

Two-thirds (67%) of the participants provided help or care to others in the last five years. Thirty-five percent reported having cared for one person, 24% for 2 to 5 people, 4% for 6 to 10 people, and 4% for more than 10 people. Females gave more help than males (73% vs. 62%), although the difference was not statistically significant. Thirty percent (40% of the males, 21% of the females) had provided care to people with HIV/AIDS. Other conditions for which many of the participants provided care included cancer (29%), muscular-skeletal illnesses (21%), cardiovascular disease (19%), and other chronic illnesses associated with the aging process (26%), e.g., visual, hearing and communication impairments. Three percent of participants reported that they had provided care to victims of LGB bias-related physical attacks.

Differences between past care recipients and non-recipients, and between past care-givers and non-givers, were examined, and the results are shown in Table 1. Those who had received help in the past were significantly older ($d = .36$, small effect size), reported worse health ($d = .66$, moderate effect size), and reported significantly more internalized homophobia ($d = .30$, small effect size) than those who had not received help. Those who had given help used more task-focused coping ($d = .49$, moderate effect size). Having received help in the past five years was strongly related to having given help in the same time period. Of those who had received caregiving, 76% had provided care to others; of those who had not received care, 60% had provided care. Although having received help in the past did not relate to willingness to help in the future, participants who had given help in the past were significantly more willing to give help again compared to those who had never helped others ($d = .57$, moderate effect size).

TABLE 1. Comparisons of Help-Recipients vs. Non-Recipients and Help-Givers vs. Non-Help Givers

Variable	Help-Recipients (n = 74)		Non-Recipients (n = 123)			Help-Givers (n = 130)		Non-Givers (n = 65)		
	M	SD	M	SD	t	M	SD	M	SD	t
Age	68.46	10.00	64.79	10.27	-2.37*	65.20	10.97	67.63	8.88	1.51
Educational level	3.97	1.67	3.61	1.70	-1.42	3.72	1.75	3.85	1.56	.50
Income	3.34	1.48	3.36	1.61	.11	3.24	1.48	3.53	1.67	1.21
Health status	3.58	.74	4.04	.66	4.53**	3.85	.75	3.94	.66	.84
Mental health status	4.04	.75	3.96	.71	-.76	4.01	.72	3.95	.74	-.49
Internalized homophobia	1.77	.58	1.61	.50	1.96*	1.66	.56	1.69	.50	-.29
Loneliness	1.91	.73	1.87	.73	.39	1.88	.74	1.87	.69	.03
Social support	1.67	.71	1.64	.73	-.31	1.60	.72	1.70	.70	.89
Task-focused coping	3.33	.76	3.36	.80	-.30	3.91	.77	3.54	.75	-3.14**
Emotion-focused coping	1.99	.59	1.94	.55	-.58	1.89	.49	2.05	.66	1.76
Perceived stress	1.52	.58	1.42	.65	-1.09	1.48	.65	1.40	.58	-.85
Perceived burden	3.16	.70	3.09	.72	-.63	3.05	.65	3.25	.79	1.87
Personal gain	3.13	.65	3.29	.57	-1.67	3.31	.55	3.03	.69	2.30**
Willingness to help	2.73	.73	2.80	.73	-.60	2.91	.67	2.50	.78	3.75**

* p < .05.
** p < .01.

Willingness to Provide Care in the Future to LGB People

When asked about willingness to provide care to specific types of people, 76% said that they would provide care to gay males, 65% to lesbians, 52% to bisexual women and men, and 54% to heterosexual people. Participants were more willing to provide care to gay males and lesbians than to bisexual or heterosexual people. The sexual orientation of the recipient of future help was related to willingness to provide care. Nearly all males (93%) were willing to care for gay men, whereas about half (52%) were willing to care for lesbians, χ^2 (1, $N = 199$) = 43.85, $p < .001$. In approximately the reverse way, 95% of the females were willing to care for lesbians, but 43% would care for gay men, χ^2 (1, $N = 198$) = 58.17, $p < .001$. There were no differences between males and females in willingness to care for bisexual or heterosexual people. Interestingly, cross-sexual orientation caregiving (e.g., lesbians helping gay men) percentages were similar to the percentages of the sample willing to help bisexual and heterosexual people.

Predicting Future Willingness to Provide Caregiving to LGB People

The following variables were used to predict willingness to help other LGB people: sex, age, educational level, income, health status, and mental health status. Personal characteristics expected to be related to propensity to help included were: internalized homophobia, loneliness, social support, task-focused coping skills, and emotion-focused coping skills. Finally, perceived stress, perceived burdens of caregiving, and the perceived personal gain of caregiving were included.

Bivariate correlations were conducted relating the above variables to willingness to help. Willingness to help correlated significantly with educational level, r (183) = $-.19$, $p < .01$; task-focused coping, r (182) = $-.16$, $p < .05$; perceived burdens of caregiving, r (145) = $-.45$, $p < .01$; and perceived personal gains from caregiving, r(186) = .45, $p < .01$. Participants with less education, and who more often used task-focused coping and less emotion-focused coping were more willing to provide care, although these relationships are small in magnitude. More importantly, participants' greater willingness to help was related to lower expectations that help would be burdensome, as well as to expecting more personal gain from helping. A hierarchical linear regression analysis was then conducted using willingness to help as the dependent variable.

Three blocks of variables were entered, in the following order: background characteristics (age, educational level, income, health status, and mental health status), personal characteristics (internalized homophobia, loneliness, social support, task-focused coping, emotion-focused coping, and perceived stress), and caregiving experiences and attitudes (having received help or not, having given help or not, perceiving burden of caregiving, and perceived gain). The first block, background characteristics, yielded a significant finding, $R^2 = .138$, $F (5, 103) = 3.30$, $p < .01$. The second block, personal characteristics, did not make a significant additional contribution to predicting willingness to help, $R^2 = .161$, $F (6, 97) = .44$, *ns*. On the other hand, adding caregiving experiences and attitudes resulted in a significant increment in R^2, $F (4, 93) = 11.89$, $p < .001$. After the addition of the third block, the final R^2 was .445 (adjusted $R^2 = .355$).

The analysis was conducted again deleting the second block of variables as it did not contribute to increased prediction. For the two-block model, R^2 was .114, $F (5, 118) = 3.03$, $p < .05$, for the demographic variables, and the addition of the caregiving variables resulted in a final R^2 of .369 (adjusted $R^2 = .319$), a significant increment, $F (4, 114) = 11.54$, $p < .001$. The caregiving experience variables added 26% ($\Delta R^2 = .255$) of the variance to the prediction based on demographic characteristics alone. The *B* coefficients, the *SE*'s and the β for the final two-block model appear in Table 2. These analyses suggest that more highly educated participants were less willing to provide help to an older LGB person, and that those who expected caregiving to be less burdensome and as more personally rewarding were more willing to help.

DISCUSSION

With few exceptions, most heterosexual older adults know the social context in which they will develop during older adulthood. This is not as predictable for today's older LGB adults. They may be isolated, having limited contact with the older LGB community, and therefore think that society's stereotypes and biases toward LGB people will dictate an aging life characterized by loneliness and illness, without much quality. Therefore, the special problems older LGB people face, including who will provide care for them, are primarily due to social and institutional biases against same-sex sexual orientation rather than to deficiencies in their families (Fullmer, 1995). This leaves the individual wondering who will replace biological family members in providing care. It also

TABLE 2. Predictors of Willingness to Provide Caregiving to Older LGB People

Variable	B	SE	β
Step 1			
Age	−.005	.006	−.09
Educational level	−.115	.038	−2.84**
Income	−.026	.041	−.059
Health status	.030	.096	.028
Mental health status	.116	.089	.117
Step 2			
Age	−.001	.005	−.015
Educational level	−.074	.033	−.182*
Income	−.027	.036	−.006
Health status	.020	.087	.019
Mental health status	.095	.078	.096
Perceived burden	−.551	.139	−.330***
Personal gain	.278	.092	.264**
Received/not received help	.000	.112	.000
Gave/not given help	.160	.113	.113

* $p < .05.$
** $p < .01.$
*** $p < .001.$

challenges LGB communities, which are faced with the question of who will provide care for their aging members. Our effort to determine characteristics of those individuals in the LGB communities who would be willing to provide care or help is useful in this regard.

LGB people share the health-related concerns of all older adults (e.g., increased incidence of chronic diseases, use of multiple medications, health-care costs not covered by insurance). Thomas (1996) noted that their situations are more complex for two reasons. First, they confront unique psychological barriers (e.g., perceived homophobia and heterosexism) and financial barriers related to health care access (e.g., no coverage on partner's health plan). Second, there are medical conditions that are particular threats for older LGB adults (e.g., cancer, anal gonorrhea, HIV/AIDS). Additionally, caregiving and care receiving are complicated because many older LGB adults have not disclosed their sexual orientation to their children or parents. For example, if one partner needs care, she or he may be separated from a life-partner and relocated to the home of a child or to an assisted living facility (Brotman et al., 2003).

Or, both partners hide their relationship in their own home if one decides to take in an ailing parent.

Caregiving

The results of this study indicate that the participants created networks that embrace caregiving in a community that is unique and whose caregiving norms vary from the traditional ones of heterosexual communities. There was a history of caregiving in the sample, with more than two-thirds having provided care in the last five years, with more than a third giving care to one person, and approximately another third providing care to from 2 to 10 people. Females gave more help than males, although the difference was not statistically significant. This varies from the pattern in the heterosexual community, where females give significantly more care than males (Canican & Oliker, 2000). The difference may not be significant among the participants in this sample because both females and males see themselves as members of a unique older adult minority community and that perception is greater than the difference between them when someone is old and ill. Also, the allocation of gender role behaviors among LGB adults is not as rigid as they are among heterosexuals (Kurdek, 1993). Additionally, the incidents of HIV/AIDS in the lesbian and gay community called on many men to provide care for partners, lovers, and friends. Forty percent of the males in the sample indicated they had provided care to individuals with this disease.

The issue of reciprocity was also an important factor to those providing care. Having received help in the past five years was strongly related to having given help in the same period. Not having traditional kin to depend on when they need help, the participants in this study "know" that providing care is an investment in receiving care when one needs it. Exchange theory provides one possible interpretation of this finding, suggesting that parties to an exchange relationship attempt to maintain balance in costs and rewards (Clark & Mills, 1993).

Care Receiving

Although slightly more than a third of the participants reported receiving help or care at least once, some indicated receiving help multiple times. Those participants who received help in the past five years were significantly older, reported worse health, and reported significantly more internalized homophobia. These results are not surprising. Chronic diseases associated with the aging process tend to increase as people get older.

Those participants who were older spent more of their lives growing up when homosexuality was classified as a mental illness in the Diagnostic and Statistical Manual of Mental Disorders; consequently, it is not surprising that they have more internalized homophobia.

Willingness to Provide Care in the Future to LGB People

More than three-fourths of the participants were willing to provide care to LGB people in the future. The sexual orientation of the recipient of future care was related to how gay men and lesbians expressed willingness to provide help. While nearly all males were willing to care for gay men, nearly all of the females were willing to care for lesbians. About half of the gay men were willing to provide care for lesbians, and almost half of the lesbians were willing to provide care for gay men. There were no differences in their willingness to provide care for bisexual or heterosexual people. As only 9% of the participants identified as bisexual, these findings were to be expected with gay men having attractions to men and lesbians having attractions to women. Also, in our gendered society, both sexes would be more comfortable in providing care that may involve touching and toileting to members of their own gender.

It was predicted that people who had greater social support, less perceived stress, greater task-focused coping skills, and fewer burdensome past caregiving experiences would be more likely to provide care to another LGB person than individuals without these characteristics. We also expected that the older LGB adults who experienced less loneliness and less internalized homophobia would be more willing to care for another LGB person. Older LGB adults who had received care themselves and who thought that they could gain personally by providing care were also expected to be more willing to help. Unexpectedly, only three factors were related to the willingness to help: expected burden, personal gain, and educational level. Those participants willing to provide care had lower expectations that it would be burdensome, and they also expected personal rewards. These participants viewed caregiving as an opportunity for personal growth, to give back to the LGB community, and to build a caregiving network that would help them in the future. We also found that more highly educated participants were less willing to provide help to an older LGB person. Anecdotal evidence suggests that these individuals tend to manage the caregiving process versus providing direct care, a factor that requires additional investigation.

Limitations of the Study and Directions for Further Research

The participants in this study were individuals connected to the LGB community, with the large majority being well educated and having good incomes; and only perceived burdens of caregiving and expected personal gains predicted their willingness to give care. Research is especially needed to examine older LGB people who are not connected to LGB communities and who are more diverse educationally and economically. As individuals with ample resources and higher education are more likely to have access to expensive care options and greater knowledge about the formal support systems, the findings of this study may underestimate the need for caregiving among older LGB adults (Sorensen & Pinquart, 2000b). Additionally, for groups of older LGB adults with resources, their views of their social networks (such as degrees of trust, loyalty and emotional bonding) are factors that need to be examined when investigating their access to nonjudgmental and sensitive caregiving.

While recruiting individuals from organizations that provide recreation and social services to older LGB adults is practical and cost effective, it limits the study's participants to individuals who have characteristics that may not be possessed by the majority of older LGB adults who would not attend activities or receive services, such as those who do not have a similar level of acceptance of their sexual orientation or who are members of cultures that do not encourage seeking services outside of the family. Those who attend organizations for older LGB adults may also be more willing to openly confront some of society's strongest taboos about sex and gender and to feel more comfortable associating with other LGB people.

This study has limitations that not only limit the generalizability of the findings based on sample selection, but also based in the nature of the questions asked in the survey. First, the hypothetical example given to assess the willingness to provide help focuses on an example of short-term recovery from surgery, which does not assess willingness to provide care for individuals with chronic long-term caregiving situations or care for individuals with terminal illnesses. We do not know how this impacted the findings and willingness to provide care in these situations. Additionally, the participants were asked about their perceived willingness to provide care, and we do not know how similar or different their responses would be to their willingness to provide care in an actual situation Other limitations result from our attempt to limit the size of the survey to increase the sample size. Consequently, we may have captured limited information about the participants' current mental and physical health statuses by using only single-item measures.

Other areas of exploration include examining the availability of potential caregivers who have not disclosed their sexual orientation at work and who may be unable to take time off to help ill friends or partners, as these people are not considered immediate family members by their employers. More detail about caregiving might have been obtained. For instance, we do not have data on individuals who needed help but did not receive it. Also, data were not available about the type of help needed. For example, did those older LGB adults with minimal and moderate levels of impairment receive the same level of help or care, and did they receive less intensive care than those with more severe impairments? Finally, information on the number of care providers that an individual had was not collected. Therefore, we do not know if the participant giving care was the only helper or part of a group of helpers.

Many older LGB adults survive because of their connections with wider LGB communities; and the older LGB adults in this study are some of those individuals (Barker, 2004). They have experienced stigma and stress resulting from societal homophobia and heteronormativity. Studies have suggested that because of these stressors, many LGB individuals have developed enhanced coping skills in old age, i.e., competencies from early life crises surrounding coming out and developing strong friendship and support networks (Brotman et al., 2003). The challenge is to see if they and the LGB communities to which they belong can translate these strengths into resources for caregiving. Additional research, using a larger and more diversified group of older LGB adults, is needed to explore other predictors of willingness to provide care so that research-based service programs can be developed. The results of the current study not only provide a basis on which future research studies can be built, but they also point to an important program strategy–helping older LGB adults understand *both* the rewards and burdens of caregiving in both establishing and coordinating caregiving programs in LGB communities.

NOTES

1. Before, 1961, homosexuality per se was illegal in the U.S, and every state had a "sodomy law" that criminalized consensual same-sex sexual behavior between adults. In, 2003, the U.S. Supreme Court, in the *Lawrence et al. v. Texas* decision, voided the

remaining thirteen sodomy laws (No. 02-102), decided June 26, 2003; http://www. supremecourtus.gov/opinions/02pdf/02-102.pdf).

2. Many would consider individuals between 40 and 59 to be middle-aged; however, recognizing that those in this study were recruited from agencies serving older LGB adults, that some traditionally middle-age adults are in intergenerational relationships and caregivers to older LGB adults, or that some have conditions which make them identify as older LGB adults, we included them in the study.

REFERENCES

Aspinwall, L., & Taylor, S. (1997). A stitch in time: Self-regulation and proactive coping. *Psychological Bulletin, 121*, 417-436.

Barker, J. C. (2004). Lesbian aging: An agenda for social research. In G. Herdt & B. deVries (eds.), *Gay and lesbian aging: Research and future directions* (pp. 29-72). New York: Springer Publishing.

Beeler, J. A., Rawls, T. D., Herdt, G., & Cohler, B. J. (1999). The needs of older lesbians in Chicago. *Journal of Gay & Lesbian Social Services, 9*(1), 31-49.

Brotman, S., Ryan, B., & Cormier, R. (2003). The health and social service needs of gay and lesbian elders and their families in Canada. *The Gerontologist, 43*(2), 192-202.

Cahill, S., South, K., & Spade, J. (2002). *Outing age: Policy issues affecting gay, lesbian, Bisexual and transgender elders.* New York: The Policy Institute of the National Gay and Lesbian Task Force.

Canican, F. M., & Oliker, S. J. (2000). *Caring and gender.* Walnut Creek, CA: Rowan & Littlefield.

Clark, M. S., & Mills, J. (1993). The difference between communal and exchange relationships. What it is and is not. *Personality and Social Psychology Bulletin, 19*, 684-691.

Cohen, J. (1988). *Statistical power for the behavioral sciences* (2nd ed.) Hillside, NJ: Erlbaum.

Cohen, S., Karmarck, T., & Mermelstein, R. (1983). A global measure of perceived stress. *Journal of Health and Social Behavior, 24*, 385-396.

Cohen, S., & Wills, T. A. (1985). Stress, social support, and buffering. *Psychological Bulletin, 98*, 310-357.

Crystal, S., Akincigil, A., Sambamoorthi, U., Wenger, N., Fleishman, J. A., Zingmond, D. S., et al. (2003). The diverse older HIV-positive population: A national profile of economic circumstances, social support, and quality of life. *Journal of Acquired Immune Deficiency Syndrome, 33*, S76-S83.

D'Augelli, A.R., & Grossman, A.H. (2000). [Challenges & Coping: The Q&A Project]. Unpublished raw data.

D'Augelli, A. R., Grossman, A. H., Hershberger, S. L., & O'Connell, T. S. (2001). Aspects of mental health among older lesbian, gay, and bisexual adults. *Aging and Mental Health, 5*, 149-158.

Dew, M. A., Goycoolea, J. M., Stukas, A. A., Switzer, G. E., Simmons, R. G., Roth, L. H., & DiMartini, A. (1998). Temporal profiles of physical health in family members of heart transplant recipients: Predictors of health change during caregiving. *Health Psychology, 17*, 138-151.

Dorfman, R., Walters, K., Burke, P., Hardin, L. Karanik, T., Raphael, J., & Silverstein, E. (1995). Old, sad and alone: The myth of the aging homosexual. *Journal of Gerontological Social Work, 24*(2), 29-44.

Dwyer, J. W., & Coward, R. T. (Eds.) (1992). *Gender, families, and elder care.* Newbury Park, CA: Sage.

Endler, N. S., & Parker J. D. A. (1990). *Coping Inventory for Stressful Situations Manual.* North Tonawanda, NY: Multi-Health Systems.

Fredriksen, K. I. (1999). Family caregiving responsibilities among lesbians and gay men. *Social Work, 44*, 142-155.

Fullmer, E. M. (1995). Challenging biases against families of older gays and lesbians. In G. C. Smith, S. S. Tobin, E. A. Robertson-Tchabo, & P. W. Power (Eds.), *Strengthening aging families: Diversity in practice and policy* (pp. 99-119). Thousand Oaks, CA: Sage.

Given, B., Stommel, M., Collins, C., King, S., & Given, C. W. (1990). Responses of elderly spouse caregivers. *Research in Nursing and Health, 13*, 17-85.

Goode, K. T., Haley, W. E., Roth, D. L., & Ford, G. R. (1998). Predicting longitudinal changes in caregiver physical and mental health: A stress process model. *Health Psychology, 17*(2), 190-198.

Goodkin, K., Heckman, T., Siegel, K., Linsk, N., Khamis, I., Lee, D., et al. (2003). "Putting a face" on HIV infection/AIDS in older adults: A psychosocial context. *Journal of Acquired Deficiency Syndromes, 33*, S171-S184.

Grossman, A. H., D'Augelli, A. R., & O'Connell, T. S. (2001). Being lesbian, gay, bisexual, and 60 or older in North America. *Journal of Gay and Lesbian Social Services, 13*(4), 23-40.

Grossman, A. H., D'Augelli, A. R., & Hershberger, S. L. (2000). Social support networks of lesbian, gay, and bisexual adults 60 years of age and older. *Journal of Gerontology: Psychological Sciences, 55B*, P171-P179.

Harris, M. (1981). Why the gays came out of the closet. In M. Harris (Ed.), *America now* (pp. 98-115). New York: Simon and Schuster.

Harris, P. B., & Bichler, J. (1997). *Men giving care: Reflections of husbands and sons.* New York: Garland.

Hash, K. (2001). Caregiving and post-caregiving experiences of midlife and older gay men and lesbians. Unpublished doctoral dissertation, Virginia Commonwealth University.

Hayes, R. D., & DiMatteo, M. R. (1987). A short-form measure of loneliness. *Journal of Personality Assessment, 51*, 69-81.

Herdt, G., & deVries, B. (2004). Introduction. In G. Herdt & B. deVries (Eds.), *Gay and lesbian aging: Research and future directions* (pp. xi-xxii). New York: Spring Publishing.

Hooyman, N. R., & Lustbader, W. (1986). *Taking care: Supporting older people and their families.* New York: The Free Press.

Jacobs, R., Rasmussen, L., & Hohman, M. (1999). The social support needs of older lesbians, gay men, and bisexuals. *Journal of Gay and Lesbian Social Services, 9*(1), 1-30.

Kurdek, L. (1993). The allocation of household labor in gay, lesbian, and heterosexual married couples. *Journal of Social Issues, 49*(3), 127-139.

Matthews, S. H., & Rosner, T. T. (1988). Shared filial responsibility: The family as the primary caregiver. *Journal of Marriage and the Family, 50*, 185-195.

Montgomery, R. J. V., Gonyea, J. G., & Hooyman, N. R. (1985). Caregiving and the experience of subjective and objective burden. *Family Relations, 34*, 19-26.

Mullins, L. C., Johnson, D. P., & Anderson, L. (1987). Elderly social relationships with adult children and close friends and depression. *Journal of Social Behavior and Personality, 2*, 225-238.

Norris, F. H., & Kaniasty, K. (1996). Received and perceived social support in times of stress: A test of the social support deterioration deterrence model. *Journal of Personality and Social Psychology, 71*, 498-511.

Pearlin, L. I., Mullan, J. T., Semple, S. J., & Skaff, M. M. (1990). Caregiving and the stress process: An overview of concepts and their measures. *The Gerontologist, 32*, 367-374.

Pinquart, M., & Sorensen, S. (2002). Factors that promote and prevent preparation for future care needs: Perceptions of older Canadian, German, and U.S. women. *Health Care for Women International, 23*, 729-741.

Porter, M., Russell, C., & Sullivan, G. (2004). Gay, old, and poor: Service delivery to aging gay men in Inner City Sydney, Australia. *Journal of Gay & Lesbian Social Services, 16*(2), 43-57.

Quam, J. K., & Whitford, G. S. (1992). Adaptation and age-related expectations of older gay and lesbian adults. *The Gerontologist, 32*, 367-374.

Rubenstein, W. B. (1996). Lesbians, gay men, and the law. In R. C. Savin-Williams, & K. M. Cohen (Eds.), *The lives of lesbians, gays, and bisexuals: Children to adults* (pp. 331-343). Forth Worth, TX: Harcourt Brace.

Shidlo, A. (1994). Internalized homophobia: Conceptual and empirical issues in measurement. In B. Greene & G. Herek (Eds.), *Lesbian and gay psychology: Theory, research, and clinical applications*. Thousand Oaks, CA: Sage.

Sorensen, S., & Pinquart, M. (2000a). Preparation for future care needs: Styles of preparation used by older Eastern German, United States, and Canadian women. *Journal of Cross-Cultural Gerontology, 15*, 349-381.

Sorensen, S., & Pinquart, M. (2000b) Vulnerability and access to resources as predictors of preparation for future care needs in the elderly. *Journal of Aging and Health, 12*, 275-300.

Thomas, J. L. (1996). Expanding knowledge of older gay men and lesbians: Retrospect and prospect. In L. Sperry, & H. Prosen (Eds.), *Aging in the twenty-first century: A developmental perspective* (pp. 141-152). New York: Garland.

Turner, H. A., Perlin, L. I., & Mullan, J. T. (1998). Sources and determinants of social support for caregivers of persons with AIDS. *Journal of Health and Social Behavior, 39*, 137-151.

Vitaliano, P. P., Young, H. M., & Russo, J. (1991). Burden: A review of measures used among caregivers of individuals with dementia. *The Gerontologist, 31*, 67-75.

Weston, K. (1991). *Families we choose: Lesbians, gays, kinship*. New York: Columbia University Press.

Wight, R. G., LeBlanc, A. J., & Aneshensel, C. S. (1998). AIDS caregiving and health among midlife and older women. *Health Psychology, 17*, 130-137.

Zarit, S. H., Reever, K., & Bach-Peterson, J. (1980). Relatives of the impaired elderly: Correlates of feelings of burden. *The Gerontologist, 20*, 649-655.

doi:10.1300/J041v18n03_02

We Cannot Go It Alone:
The Impact of Informal Support
and Stressors in Older Gay, Lesbian
and Bisexual Caregivers

R. Andrew Shippy

SUMMARY. This study examines the effect of stressors and support resources among aging gay men and lesbian women who are caring for their families, both biological families and chosen families. Forty-five percent ($N = 155$) of the gay men and lesbians in a large study of caregiving were providing some type of caregiving assistance. Lesbian and bisexual women were twice as likely to provide caregiving to biological family, usually a parent, than gay and bisexual men. Results show that gender, strain and family expectations are predictors of greater burden for caregivers, regardless of the care recipient. However, buffering effects of support resources vary by caregiving situation; availability of support was not a significant predictor for family of origin caregivers, but the availability of emotional support predicted lower levels of burden for family of choice caregivers. These findings have implications for health and social care providers as well as public policies that need to be

R. Andrew Shippy, PhD Candidate, is affiliated with the AIDS Community Research Initiative of America, New York, NY.

[Haworth co-indexing entry note]: "We Cannot Go It Alone: The Impact of Informal Support and Stressors in Older Gay, Lesbian and Bisexual Caregivers." Shippy, R. Andrew. Co-published simultaneously in *Journal of Gay & Lesbian Social Services* (The Haworth Press, Inc.) Vol. 18, No. 3/4, 2007, pp. 39-51; and: *Caregiving with Pride* (ed: Karen I. Fredriksen-Goldsen) The Haworth Press, Inc., 2007, pp. 39-51. Single or multiple copies of this article are available for a fee from The Haworth Document Delivery Service [1-800-HAWORTH, 9:00 a.m. - 5:00 p.m. (EST). E-mail address: docdelivery@haworthpress.com].

Available online at http://jglss.haworthpress.com

doi:10.1300/J041v18n03_03

39

responsive to the unique needs of lesbians and gay men and their families. doi:10.1300/J041v18n03_03 *[Article copies available for a fee from The Haworth Document Delivery Service: 1-800-HAWORTH. E-mail address: <docdelivery@haworthpress.com> Website: <http://www.HaworthPress.com> © 2007 by The Haworth Press, Inc. All rights reserved.]*

KEYWORDS. Caregiving, informal support, stress, gay, lesbian, bisexual, family of choice, aging

INTRODUCTION

Despite the ubiquity of caregiving in today's aging society, the caregiving experiences of lesbian, gay and bisexual adults has received little attention, except in the case of AIDS caregiving (Fredriksen, 1999; Hash, 2001; Patterson, 1992). The caregiving literature is rife with examples of the negative impact of caregiving on an individual's sense of well-being (Anderson et al., 1995; Cantor, 1983; Goodman & Shippy, 2002; Schulz et al., 1995; Skaff & Pearlin, 1992; Walker et al., 1992; Zarit, Todd, & Zarit, 1986). Despite these inimical effects, research has shown that people care for loved ones for a variety of reasons, ranging from feelings of obligation and fear of institutionalization (Carter & Golant, 1994) to feelings of pride in their ability to care for loved ones in their homes (Farran, Keane-Hagerty, Sallowat, Kupferer, & Wilken, 1991).

The literature has defined negative psychological outcomes for caregivers in many ways (Schulz, O'Brien, Bookwala, & Fleissner, 1995; Stull, Kosloski, & Kercher, 1994). In this study, distress was assessed using caregivers' ratings of the burden they experienced while providing caregiving assistance to a loved one. According to the stress-process model, stressors are events or circumstances that directly or indirectly create distress causing the individual to cope with external demands and internal emotional reactions (Lazarus & Folkman, 1984).

The stress process model also posits that personal resources, like informal social support, can reduce the effect of stressors on levels of distress (Lawton, Kleban, Moss, Rovine, & Glicksman, 1989; Lazarus & Folkman, 1984; Pearlin, Mullan, Semple, & Skaff, 1990). Informal support networks can reduce emotional distress, health concerns, and economic strain (Clipp & George, 1990; Perlin, et al., 1990; Thompson, Futterman, Gallagher-Thompson, Rose, & Lovett, 1993) but also carry negative consequences (Schrimshaw & Siegel, 2003). In this study, both positive and negative aspects of informal support were examined. The basic conceptual framework was that difficulties with family and family expectations can increase stress while instrumental and emotional support can ameliorate some of the burden that lesbian, gay and bisexual caregivers experience.

In order to assess the stress-buffering effects of informal social support, a direct effects model was tested (Cohen & Wills, 1985). Informal support may affect burden, irrespective of the presence of stressors, by buttressing self-confidence and by providing concrete assistance with caregiving tasks (Krause & Borawski-Clark, 1994). Emotional and instrumental assistance may have different effects, but both should have a negative association with burden.

METHOD

Data for this study were drawn from a larger study of caregiving in the LGBT community in New York City ($N = 341$ gay, lesbian, bisexual and transgender adults over age 50). The large study was a collaborative effort of Pride Senior Network, the Policy Institute of the National Gay and Lesbian Task Force, and Fordham University Graduate School of Social Service. As is the case with most research involving the gay community, it was impossible to obtain a random sample; the current sample is purposive and not necessarily generalizable to all aging lesbian, gay and bisexual adults. (Detailed study procedures can be found in Cantor, Brennan and Shippy, 2004).

Participants

Table 1 contains a profile of the caregivers. Slightly less than half of the 341 study participants were providing some type of caregiving, including 18% ($N = 62$) who cared for a family of origin member and 23% ($N = 79$) who cared for a member of their chosen family. An additional 4% of the caregivers had provided care for both family of origin and family of choice members. Women were twice as likely as men to be family of origin caregivers chi square $(1, N = 336) = 15.28, p < .001$. This study focuses on the 155 LGBT caregivers (97 men, 57 women, and 1 caregiver who did not identify a gender) from the larger study. All the caregivers identified as gay (62%), lesbian (34%), or bisexual (4%). The average age of the caregivers was 60 years and 2/3 were White. African-American and Hispanic caregivers made up 13% and 16% of

TABLE 1. Demographic Profile of Aging Lesbian, Gay and Bisexual Caregivers

	Family of Origin (N = 75)	Family of Choice (N = 83)	Comparison
Age			$X^2 = 6.50^*$
50-59	56.0	44.6	
60-69	37.3	37.3	
70+	6.7	18.1	
Race/Ethnicity			$X^2 = 0.88$
White	67.6	70.7	
Black	13.5	8.5	
Hispanic	16.2	15.9	
Other	2.7	4.9	
Relationship Status			$X^2 = 4.77$
Single	59.5	45.7	
Partnered	32.9	44.4	
Divorced/Separated	15.1	9.8	
Living arrangement			$X^2 = 0.72$
Alone	52.1	50.6	
With partner	32.9	37.0	
With others	15.1	12.3	
Self-Rated Health			$X^2 = 0.90$
Excellent/Good	48.6	43.9	
Fair	40.5	46.3	
Poor	10.8	9.8	
Education			$X^2 = 6.06$
Less than high school	6.8	8.5	
High school graduate	12.2	11.0	
Some college	16.2	17.1	
College graduate	12.2	23.2	
Graduate school	52.7	40.2	
Employment			$X^2 = 14.33^*$
Working full-time	43.2	34.1	
Working part-time	10.8	6.1	
Self-employed	9.5	17.1	
Retired	24.3	39.0	
Unemployed	4.1	2.4	
Other	8.1	1.2	
Income Level			$X^2 = 7.35$
<$10,000	4.2	7.6	
$10,001-$25,000	16.9	13.9	
$25,001-$50,000	32.4	35.4	
$50,001-$100,000	39.4	30.4	
$100,001-$150,000	7.0	6.3	
$150,001+	0.0	6.3	

the sample, while the remaining 4% were Asian or some other race. Ninety percent of caregivers reported at least fair health and an equal proportion had at least a high school diploma (66% had college and/or graduate degrees).

Instrument

The survey instrument consisted of four separate sections comprised of several standard measures and additional questions drawn from previous LGBT studies as well as studies of caregiving and social networks that were germane to this study. The first and last sections consisted of basic demographic information and participants' personal needs, including availability of informal social support, network composition and several other demographic questions.

Sections 2 and 3 were identical sections that contained questions about caregiving to assess two different caregiving situations: caring for biological family members and for non-kin. Section 2 dealt with family members, defined for this study as anyone from the respondent's biological family (e.g., parent, child, etc.). Section 3 dealt with non-family members (e.g., partner, spouse, friend, etc.). The reasoning behind this sensitive decision to exclude partners and spouses from their usual place as "family members" was to examine in detail the extent to which LGBT elders care for biological family and/or chosen family members. Items included the type and extent of caregiving assistance, amount of time devoted to caregiving, difficulties with the care recipient's family, family expectations and items that measured the emotional, financial, and physical strain of caregiving as well as caregiver burden.

Strain was measured by three separate items measured on a 5-point Likert-type scale (1 = Little or None, 5 = A great deal). The three items' scores were summed to produce a strain index, ranging from 3-15. The caregiving burden index comprised 12 dichotomous (i.e., yes/no) items that assessed various aspects of caregiving (e.g., caregiving limits my social life, my caregiving responsibilities have forced me to come out [as an LGBT person]). Single items were used to assess difficulty with family members and whether the caregiver's sexual orientation caused family members to have different expectations regarding caregiving. Two separate 4-level Likert-type items were used to measure the level of instrumental and emotional support available for caregivers (1 = most of the time, 4 = not at all).

FINDINGS

Family of Origin Caregivers

The majority of family of origin caregivers were caring for a parent (84%), while 4% were caring for a child, 7% were caring for a sibling and 5% were caring for another member of their family of origin. A minority of family of origin caregivers (26%) lived with the care recipient. The types of assistance most often provided to care recipients reflect this living arrangement. Forty percent of the caregivers felt that the most important function was providing emotional support, while 39% said that case management (e.g., making arrangements for medical care, intervene with doctors or social workers, making financial decisions) was the most important type of assistance they provided. Since most of these caregivers did not live with the care recipient, it is not surprising that personal or household care were not identified as frequently as other types of assistance.

Although most caregivers did not live with those receiving care, the majority (71%), of them were involved at least several times a week and devoted an average of 29 hours per week to their caregiving responsibilities. One reason that caregivers were so involved was that many had sole (37%) or primary (30%) responsibility for the care recipient.

It is not uncommon in family caregiving for there to be tension, particularly among siblings when caring for an elderly parent. The caregivers in this study were no exception: 33% reported experiencing some type of difficulties with the care recipient's family and friends. For lesbian, gay, and bisexual adults, their sexual orientation may unfortunately become a source of contention for some family members. Approximately one-third (34%) of caregivers stated that their families expected more of them because of their sexual orientation. One explanation for this expectation was that the caregiver did not have explicit "family" obligations, such as children or a spouse (even if they had a partner), like their heterosexual siblings.

There were no gender differences in the amount of time spent in caregiving activities (hours/week) or level of strain (emotional, physical, or financial) experienced, but women reported greater caregiving burden than men ($t(72) = -2.43, p < .05$). Women who were caring for a member of their family of origin were significantly more likely to take time off work, conceal their sexual orientation, and experience strained relationships with their partners than men (Table 2).

TABLE 2. Comparison of Sex Differences Within Family of Origin and Family of Choice Caregivers

	Family of Origin (N = 75)			Family of Choice (N = 83)		
	Male	Female		Male	Female	
Caregiver (%)	15.9	35.9	$X^2 = 16.71^{**}$	26.2	20.4	$X^2 = 1.30$
Hours/week (M)	23.6	34.3	$t = -1.21$	43.8	54.1	$t = -0.86$
Strain (M)	8.0	8.8	$t = -1.22$	7.4	8.1	$t = -1.07$
Time off work (%)	43.2	70.3	$X^2 = 5.51^*$	31.3	62.5	$X^2 = 7.17^{**}$
Hide orientation (%)	2.7	24.3	$X^2 = 7.40^{**}$	9.0	25.0	$X^2 = 3.97^*$
Strain partner relationship (%)	8.1	37.8	$X^2 = 9.24^{**}$	9.0	20.8	$X^2 = 2.35$
Limits social life (%)	59.5	70.3	$X^2 = 0.95$	41.8	66.7	$X^2 = 4.38^*$

Family of Choice Caregivers

The lesbian, gay, and bisexual adults who were caring for a member of their family of choice cared for partners (53%) and friends (34%). An additional 13% cared for individuals whose relationship was not specified. Given the historical devastation of the gay community by HIV/ AIDS, it is not a surprise that 41% of the family of choice caregivers were caring for someone who was living with HIV/AIDS. However, the other 59% of caregivers were providing care for essentially the same types of illnesses found in older adults. Family of choice caregivers were more likely to care for someone of the same gender than traditional caregivers. Eighty-five percent of the women cared for a woman, while 94% of the men provided care to a man.

Family of choice caregivers were more likely to live with the care recipient (54% versus 26%) than those caring for a member of their family of origin. Nearly all of the family of choice caregivers always or often provided emotional support. Over three-quarters of these caregivers provided household help (e.g., doing laundry and shopping) and over half (55%) cooked always or often, types of assistance typical of a caregiver who lives with the care recipient. Also indicative of the intensity of the caregiving situation was the level of hands-on personal care. Forty percent of the caregivers were regularly involved in bathing and grooming the care recipient. The majority of caregivers were routinely involved in decision-making (54%) and case management tasks (66%).

Family of choice caregivers also answered questions about the stress they experience as caregivers. Not surprisingly, 81% of caregivers said they were involved in frequent assistance (daily or several times weekly), with an average of 46 hours in a typical week. Two-thirds of the caregivers were either sole (43%) or primary (25%) caregivers. Use of formal care providers was low, but a significant minority of the family of choice providers (26%) had difficulties with formal care providers during the caregiving episode. Caregivers said that stigma and fear of discrimination because of their sexual orientation influenced caregivers' relations with medical personnel, but reported fewer conflicts with social workers.

There were no gender differences in the level of strain (emotional, physical, or financial) experienced or number of hours involved in caregiving each week, but women again reported greater caregiving burden than men during the course of providing care to family of choice, ($t(84) = -2.10, p < .05$). Female family of choice caregivers were more likely to take time off work, conceal their sexual orientation, and report that their caregiving responsibilities limit their social life than male caregivers (Table 2).

PREDICTORS OF CAREGIVER BURDEN

The means and standard deviations of the key variables used in the regression models are found in Table 3. Bivariate analyses of key study variables revealed that caregiver burden was consistently related to study variables across both caregiving conditions (Table 4). Caregiver burden was positively related to being female, confrontations with family members, family members' expectations because of one's sexual orientation, and higher levels of strain. Caregiver burden was negatively related to higher level of support availability.

Table 5 presents two hierarchical multiple regression analyses of caregiver burden on demographic variables, stressors, and support variables for aging lesbian, gay and bisexual caregivers. Demographic variables were entered first, followed by stressors. The final block consisted of measures of informal support availability, both instrumental and emotional assistance were included.

The regression model was significant, ($F(8, 61) = 8.00, p < .01$) and accounted for 51% of the variance in caregiver burden among family of origin caregivers. Three of the variables were significant predictors of caregiver burden: sex, family expectations and strain. Burden is higher

TABLE 3. Comparison of Key Variables Among Family of Origin and Family of Choice Caregivers

	Family of Origin (N = 75)		Family of Choice (N = 83)	
	M	(SD)	M	(SD)
Caregiver demographics				
Sex	1.50	.50	1.26	.44
Race (white)	.68	.47	.71	.46
Education	4.92	1.34	4.73	1.38
Stressors				
Family problems	.32	.47	.24	.43
Family expectations	.39	.49	.39	.49
Strain	8.37	2.75	7.61	2.80
Support				
Instrumental support	1.96	1.05	1.99	.97
Emotional support	1.69	.88	1.65	.85

Note. Sex (1 = male, 2 = female); Race (1 = white, 2 = non-white); Education (1 = elementary or less, 6 = graduate school); Family problems (0 = no, 1 = yes); Family expectations (1 = family expected more/less of me because of my sexual orientation, 0 = no differences); Strain (3 = little/no strain, 15 = great deal of strain); Instrumental support (1 = most of the time, 4 = not at all); Emotional support (1 = most of the time, 4 = not at all)

TABLE 4. Correlation Matrix of Key Variables

	1	2	3	4	5	6	7	8	9
1. sex		−.21	−.24*	−.12	.05	.07	−.01	.12	.26*
2. race	−.19		.34**	−.19	.30*	.22	.10	−.08	−.11
3. education	−.25*	.49**		−.13	.39**	−.03	−.06	−.25*	−.31**
4. family problems	.03	−.17	−.06		.09	−.11	−.03	−.01	−.26*
5. family expectations	−.08	.38**	.37**	.12		.06	.03	−.15	−.29*
6. strain	−.13	.22	.11	−.34**	.05		−.07	−.04	.44**
7. instrumental support	−.02	−.01	−.03	−.19	−.12	.23*		.68**	.03
8. emotional support	.02	−.16	−.32**	−.04	−.35**	.08	.34**		.22
9. burden	.24*	−.14	−.30**	−.39**	−.46**	.41**	.41**	.42**	

Note. Correlations normal type represent family of origin caregivers, those in **bold type** represent family of choice caregivers.

TABLE 5. Hierarchical Multiple Regression of Caregiver Burden for Lesbian, Gay and Bisexual Family of Origin and Family of Choice Caregivers

	Family of Origin (N = 75)		Family of Choice (N = 83)	
	B	(SE)	B	(SE)
Caregiver demographics				
Sex	.997*	.503	.973*	.492
Race (white)	.098	.581	.080	.552
Education	.012	.230	−.227	.185
Stressors				
Family problems	.158	.567	.737	.553
Family expectations	1.496**	.569	1.451**	.492
Strain	.540**	.095	.393**	.082
Support				
Instrumental support	−.154	.319	.359	.251
Emotional support	.378	.389	.653*	.294
Final R^2	.512		.616	

among females, people whose family expect them to do more because of their sexual orientation (not having traditional "family" commitments), and people who reported greater levels of physical, emotional and financial strain.

The regression model for family of choice caregivers was also significant, $(F(8, 67) = 13.43, p < .01)$, accounting for a total of 62% of the variance in caregiver burden. Again, females, people whose family expect them to do more, and people who experienced greater levels of strain reported higher levels of burden. In addition, caregivers without readily available emotional support reported higher levels of burden (Table 5).

DISCUSSION

This study demonstrates that lesbian, gay and bisexual caregivers may face not only the burdens of caregiving, but perceived stigma and discrimination as well. Depending on the caregiving situation, social support may not significantly affect the level of burden that lesbian, gay and bisexual caregivers experience. For family of origin caregivers, the availability of instrumental and emotional support from informal social networks did not significantly affect assessments of caregiver burden, but emotional support was a significant, positive predictor for family of choice caregivers. While seemingly counterintuitive, it is possible that the extent of caregiving responsibilities, in the context of not living with the care recipient, outweighed the influence of social support. It is also possible that the difficulties with family members, particularly siblings in the context of caring for a biological family member, mitigated the effect of informal social support.

The study offers concrete evidence that, contrary to popular beliefs, lesbian, gay and bisexual older adults are not estranged from their biological families. The fact that two-thirds of the caregivers' families did not have different expectations of them because of their sexual orientation underscores family involvement and acceptance. The findings also support earlier research by Fredriksen (1999) that also demonstrated that gay and lesbian adults are deeply involved in family caregiving responsibilities. In fact, these individuals are an integral component of the 26 million informal caregivers in the United States. These caregivers are dedicated to and involved with both families of origin and families of choice. Despite the fact that many lesbian, gay and bisexual adults are caring for parents, siblings, children and partners, they may not be afforded the same access to social, medical and financial care resources that are accessed by other caregivers. These caregivers are highly dedicated and like so many other caregivers, they need access to these resources to continue to provide much needed assistance to loved ones.

These analyses demonstrate that lesbian, gay and bisexual caregivers are affected by the same types of stressors that all caregivers must face. The fact that women experienced more burden reinforces the similarities of this study population and the general population more than illustrating differences in the experience itself. Women are often called upon to provide caregiving, especially for their parents. They are frequently required to negotiate their own family's needs and work responsibilities in the course of caring for a parent, child, partner or friend. However, it is important to note that the male caregivers in this study were also involved in intensive caregiving duties. Unlike much of the caregiving literature that reports men are less involved in caregiving than female relatives, both gay men and lesbian women provided as much or more assistance than their family members. In fact, many of the caregivers were solely responsible for the care of their other family member. Unlike other caregivers, however, the sexual orientation of a significant group of the caregivers caused difficulties with both family and formal care providers. Caregivers in this study have suggested that the LGBT community has a role in caring for its older members, reflecting ever-present stigma and lack of sensitivity in mainstream health and social welfare services.

There were some limitations that should be carefully addressed in future research. The sample, drawn from members of LGBT organizations in New York City, did not represent the full racial/ethnic, religious and economic diversity of the LGBT communities in New York City. The cross-sectional design limited perceptions of stress and burden, while a longitudinal design would be better able to assess family changes and development of coping strategies over time. These limits notwithstanding, this study provides evidence that gay and lesbian individuals are deeply involved in caring for their biological and chosen families. Health and social care providers must be aware of and sensitive to the unique needs of these caregivers. We must all become advocates for change in existing and future policy that is not inclusive of the needs of lesbian, gay and bisexual caregivers.

REFERENCES

Anderson, C. S., Linto, J., & Stewart-Wynne, E. G. (1995). A population-based assessment of the impact and burden of caregiving for long-term stroke survivors. *Stroke, 26,* 843-849.

Brody, E. M. (1985). Parent care as a normative family stress. *The Gerontologist, 25,* 19-29.

Cantor, M.H. (1983). Strain among caregivers: A study of the experiences in the United States. *The Gerontologist, 23,* 597-624.

Cantor, M. H., Brennan, M., & Shippy, R. A. (2004). *Caregiving among older lesbian, gay, bisexual, and transgender New Yorkers.* New York: National Gay and Lesbian Task Force Policy Institute.

Carter, R., & Golant, K. (1994). Helping yourself help others: A book for caregivers. New York: Random House.

Clipp, E. C., & George, L. K. (1990). Caregiver needs and patterns of social support. *Journal of Gerontology: Social Sciences, 45,* S102-S111.

Cohen, S., & Wills, T. A. (1985). Stress, social support, and the buffering hypothesis. *Psychological Bulletin, 98,* 310-335.

Farran, C. J., Keane-Hagerty, E., Sallowat, S., Kupferer, S., & Wilken, C. S. (1991). Finding meaning: An alternative paradigm for Alzheimer's Disease family caregivers. *The Gerontologist, 31*(4), 483-489.

Fredriksen, K. I. (1999). Family caregiving responsibilities among lesbians and gay men. *Social Work, 44*(2), 142-155.

Goodman, C. R., & Shippy, R. A. (2002). Is It Contagious? Affect Similarity among Spouses. *Aging & Mental Health, 6*(3), 266-274.

Hash, K. M. (2002). Preliminary study of caregiving and post-caregiving experiences of older gay men and lesbians. *Journal of Gay and Lesbian Social Services, 13*(4), 87-94.

Krause, N., & Borawski-Clark, E. (1994). Clarifying the functions of social support in later life. *Research on Aging, 16*, 251-279.

Lawton, M. P., Kleban, M. H., Moss, M., Rovine, M., & Glicksman, A. (1989). Measuring caregiving appraisal. *Journal of Gerontology: Psychological Sciences, 44*, P61-P71.

Lazarus, R. S., & Folkman, S. (1984). *Stress appraisal and coping.* New York: Springer.

Patterson, C. J. (1992). Children of gay and lesbian parents. *Child Development, 63*, 1025-1042.

Pearlin, L. I., Mullan, J. T., Semple, S. J., & Skaff, M. M. (1990). Caregiving and the stress process: An overview of concepts and their measures. *The Gerontologist, 30*, 583-594.

Schrimshaw, E. W., & Siegel, K. (2003). Perceived Barriers to Social Support from Family and Friends among Older Adults with HIV/AIDS. *Journal of Health Psychology, 8, 738-752.*

Schulz, R., O'Brien, A. T., Bookwala, J., & Fleissner, K. (1995). Psychiatric and physical morbidity effects in Alzheimer's disease caregiving: Prevalence, correlates, and causes. *The Gerontologist, 35*, 771-791.

Skaff, M. M., & Pearlin, L. I. (1992). Caregiving: Role engulfment and the loss of self. *The Gerontologist, 32*, 656-664.

Stull, D. E., Kosloski, K., & Kercher, K. (1994). Caregiver burden and generic well-being: Opposite sides of the same coin? *The Gerontologist, 34*, 88-94.

Thompson, E. H., Futterman, A. M., Gallagher-Thompson, D., Rose, J. M., & Lovett, S. B. (1993). Social support and caregiving burden in family caregivers of frail elders. *Journal of Gerontology: Social Sciences, 48*, S245-S254.

Walker, A. J., Martin, S. S. K., & Jones, L. L. (1992). The benefit and costs of caregiving and care receiving for daughters and mothers. *Journal of Gerontology, 47*, S130-S139.

Zarit, S. H., Todd, P. A., & Zarit, J. M. (1986). Subjective burden of husbands and wives as caregivers: A longitudinal study. *The Gerontologist, 23*(3), 260-266.

doi:10.1300/J041v18n03_03

HIV/AIDS Caregiving:
Predictors of Well-Being and Distress

Karen I. Fredriksen-Goldsen

SUMMARY. HIV/AIDS continues to be a serious public health issue. As HIV changes from an acute disease to a more chronic illness, it places increased responsibility on family caregivers to provide on-going assistance. Based on a conceptual model of caregiving resilience, this study found high variation in caregiving outcomes with many caregivers demonstrating high levels of well-being despite adverse life circumstances. Factors that contributed significantly to caregiver well-being included income, caregiver health, discrimination, multiple loss, dispositional optimism and self-empowerment. These findings suggest that HIV/AIDS and caregiving entail more than stress and distress and that future research needs to consider caregiving within the context of a historically disadvantaged community, resilience of informal caregivers, and risk and protective factors at the personal, cultural and community levels. Such information is necessary to design community-based interventions to support informal caregivers and persons living with HIV/AIDS. doi:10.1300/J041v18n03_04 *[Article copies available for a fee from The Haworth Document Delivery Service: 1-800-HAWORTH. E-mail address:*

Karen I. Fredriksen-Goldsen, PhD, is Associate Professor and Director, Institute for Multigenerational Health, School of Social Work, University of Washington, 4101 15th Avenue NE, Seattle, WA 98195.

[Haworth co-indexing entry note]: "HIV/AIDS Caregiving: Predictors of Well-Being and Distress." Fredriksen-Goldsen, Karen I. Co-published simultaneously in *Journal of Gay & Lesbian Social Services* (The Haworth Press, Inc.) Vol. 18, No. 3/4, 2007, pp. 53-73; and: *Caregiving with Pride* (ed: Karen I. Fredriksen-Goldsen) The Haworth Press, Inc., 2007, pp. 53-73. Single or multiple copies of this article are available for a fee from The Haworth Document Delivery Service [1-800-HAWORTH, 9:00 a.m. - 5:00 p.m. (EST). E-mail address: docdelivery@haworthpress.com].

KEYWORDS. Caregiving, family, care, resiliency, resilience, well-being, distress

INTRODUCTION

HIV/AIDS continues to be a serious public health problem on both national and international levels. The number of people living with HIV in the world today has increased to approximately 38 million people (UNAIDS, 2004). In the U.S. gay and bisexual men still constitute one of the groups with the highest rate of AIDS, although there are significant changes in prevalence rates as increasing numbers of persons are exposed through intravenous drug use and heterosexual contact (Centers for Disease Control and Prevention, 2003). Among the nearly 300,000 adult and adolescent (thirteen or older) U.S. males living with AIDS, approximately 58% are men who have sex with men, 8% are men who have sex with men and are also injection drug users, 23% are injection-drug users only, and 10% are exposed through heterosexual contact (Centers for Disease Control and Prevention, 2003).

Given medical advances, such as antiretroviral therapies (ART), the nature and progression of HIV in the U.S. has changed dramatically from an acute to a more chronic condition. Recent public health data demonstrate a slowing of declines in new AIDS cases, continued declines in AIDS-related deaths, and increases in the numbers of persons living with AIDS (Center for Disease Control and Prevention, 2003). Concomitantly, there has been a shift from hospital-based care to more extensive use of community and home-based assistance. These changes have placed added responsibility on informal caregivers to provide ongoing assistance to people living with HIV/AIDS.

To date, the vast majority of caregiving research has examined the experiences of family caregivers providing assistance to older adults with other chronic conditions, with more limited attention to HIV/AIDS-related caregiving. HIV/AIDS care is unique in several respects, including the prevalence of care for younger care recipients and younger caregivers (Nimmons, 2002; Sipes, 1998; Turner & Catania, 1997), the risk of HIV/AIDS among stigmatized groups, and the caregiver's potential self-identification with the disease (Sipes, 2002; Wight, 2000; Wight, 2002).

Caregiver distress has been described as the secondary epidemic associated with the HIV/AIDS crisis (Rait, 1991). Caregiving has been found to adversely affect the psychological well-being of informal caregivers (Pearlin et al., 1994; Irving, Bor, & Catalan, 1995; Tolliver, 2001) and to result in the restriction of opportunities for personal, social and economic development (Callery, 2000; Clipp et al., 1995; Turner et al., 1994). Informal caregivers to persons with HIV/AIDS report experiencing problems with economic burden as a result of their care responsibilities (Raveis & Siegel, 1991; Wight, 2000).

Stress and coping theory has been extensively utilized in caregiving research and the primary focus has been on how stress results in distress (Sipes, 2002; Wight, 2002). Yet, HIV/AIDS caregivers also report salutary consequences associated with the provision of care (Callery, 2000) and their ability to create meaning out of adverse life circumstances (Folkman et al., 1994b; Poindexter, 2001; Tolliver, 2001). HIV/AIDS caregivers have reported a sense of personal growth resulting from their care responsibilities as well as the enhancement of intimacy between the caregiver and care recipient (Clipp et al., 1995; Cowles & Rodgers, 1994; Folkman et al., 1994b; Poindexter, 2001; Tolliver, 2001).

While positive gains from HIV/AIDS caregiving have been explored, research has not adequately examined the predictors of caregiver well-being or the relationship between positive and negative outcomes and the possibility that physical and psychological well-being can co-exist with distress produced by high or moderately high adverse life circumstances. This study is designed to address these gaps and address the following research questions: In this study what are the background characteristics and care responsibilities of informal caregivers assisting gay men living with HIV/AIDS? What background characteristics and risk and protective factors predict caregiver distress and well-being? Such information is central to developing effective culturally appropriate interventions to support informal caregivers and persons living with HIV/AIDS.

CONCEPTUAL FRAMEWORK

By relying on stress and coping models, the primary focus in caregiving research has been on how individual characteristics and coping processes interact with stress and result in burden and distress. Resilience as a conceptual framework is relevant to understanding how families' capabilities can buffer them from the disruptions of excessive demands

(Walsh, 1996, 1998, 2002). For example, the Resiliency Model of Family Stress, Adjustment and Adaptation (McCubbin & McCubbin, 1993) has been applied when families face chronic strain and heavy demands within the family system, e.g., family care of children with physical disabilities (Robinson, 1997), chronic illness (Garwick, Koohrman, Titus, Wolman & Blum, 1999; Svavarsdottir, McCubbin & Kane, 2000), and mental illness (Rungreangkulkij & Gillis, 2000) as well as the care of adults with mental retardation (Lustig, 1999) and HIV/AIDS (Fredriksen-Goldsen, 2003; Thompson, 1999).

Resilience is defined here as the behavioral patterns, functional competence and cultural capacities that individuals, families and communities utilize under adverse circumstances, and the ability to integrate adversity as a catalyst for growth and development. As noted by Ryff, Keyes, and Hughes (2003), some individuals are resilient because of adversity, not despite adversity. Thus, a conceptual model of caregiving resilience is applicable for examining caregiving processes and outcomes within historically disadvantaged communities, such as among gay men living with HIV/AIDS and their informal caregivers. Four factors are salient: (1) *Background characteristics*; (2) *Risk factors*; (3) *Protective factors*; and, (4) *Caregiving outcomes*. The conceptual framework is illustrated in Figure 1 and described below.

FIGURE 1. The Caregiving Resilience Model

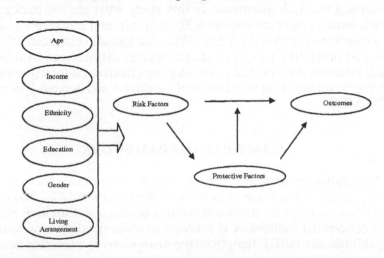

Background characteristics: Individual background factors influence how people manage adversity and risk within the context of their family, community and culture. Theoretically relevant background characteristics of HIV/AIDS caregivers–e.g., age, gender, ethnicity, income and education–are expected to impact caregiving outcomes. To date, relatively little is known about how the background characteristics of HIV/AIDS caregivers impact risk and protective factors and variations in caregiving outcomes, especially caregiver well-being.

Risk factors: This study examined the outcomes experienced by HIV/AIDS caregivers and their exposure to risk (Patterson, 2002). Risk factors incorporate the adversity (suffering, affliction or misfortune [Gove, 1993]) in people's lives, including those related to caregiving as well as those impacting historically disadvantaged communities. The following components of caregiving risk were examined: (1) health condition of the care recipient and caregiver, (2) functional and cognitive impairment levels of the care recipient, (3) hours of care provided, (4) caregiving strain, and (5) conflict in the caregiver's social network. In addition, risk factors associated with living within historically disadvantaged communities will also be examined, including (6) discrimination and (7) multiple loss. Risk factors are predicted to impact caregiver outcomes, with increased risk resulting in increased levels of distress and decreased levels of well-being. In the general caregiving literature relatively little is known about how potential risk factors impacting historically disadvantaged communities (such as discrimination and multiple loss) may influence caregiving outcomes.

Protective factors: Caregivers are active in the process of adapting and integrating their experiences when providing care. Protective factors emerge within individual, familial, cultural, and community contexts and are the capacities that are utilized to buffer risk. In this study several protective factors have been identified, which may serve a protective function for caregivers within historically disadvantaged communities, including caregiver optimism, spiritual orientation, empowerment and social support. It is hypothesized that these protective factors will be associated with decreased caregiver distress and increased well-being.

Caregiving outcomes: HIV/AIDS caregiving has repeatedly been found to be significantly associated with increased levels of caregiver burden and distress (Callery, 2000; Turner & Catania, 1997; Wight, 2000, 2002; Wight, LeBlanc & Aneshenesel, 1998). To date, less is known about caregiver well-being. In most previous research well-being is defined by the absence or lower levels of other types of psychological distress. The lack of conceptual clarity between caregiving distress and well-being likely underlies the inadequate attention to variations in caregiving outcomes. In this study we will examine both caregiver distress and well-being.

METHODS

Sample

The data used in this analysis is drawn from a larger study of 154 pairs of informal HIV/AIDS caregivers and their care recipients living in a large urban area. A caregiver is defined as a partner or other family member, friend or neighbor who provides unpaid assistance, such as personal care, providing or arranging housekeeping or transportation, assisting with financial matters or providing emotional support, to a self-identified gay man living with a confirmed AIDS diagnosis.

The caregivers were recruited using multiple sources and contacted via announcements regarding the study at various health, human service and community based organizations as well as in community based newspapers and newsletters (e.g., HIV/AIDS-related health clinics and support groups, buddy programs serving people with HIV/AIDS, and community based churches and social groups). Recruiting from a number of sites minimized biases as compared to relying on a sample drawn solely from health clinics.

Face to face interviews were conducted by graduate students in the social and behavioral sciences with experience working with HIV/AIDS populations. The interviews lasted 60-90 minutes, and the caregivers and their care recipients were interviewed in separate rooms, but simultaneously to insure that members of the dyad did not influence each other's responses. The interviews were conducted at a time and location of the caregiver and care recipient's choice, provided that privacy could be insured. Each caregiver and care recipient received a $20.00 honorarium for participating in the interview. The data collected were entered on standardized forms as well as notes on the interview protocol. Confidentiality was maintained throughout all phases of data gathering and analysis.

Caregivers of gay men with HIV/AIDS are the primary focus of this study for two reasons. First, gay men constitute one of the groups with the highest rate of HIV/AIDS in the U.S. Second, the risk and protective factors impacting these caregivers may differ from other groups given the stigmatized nature of HIV/AIDS care and same-sex sexual contact.

Measures

In addition to the socio-demographic and background variables included in the model (such as age, income, gender, ethnicity and education), the other theoretically relevant variables were operationalized as follows:

Risk factors: Care recipient health status was measured by the Physical Self Maintenance Scale (PSMS), Instrumental Activities of Daily Living Scale (IADL), and the Neuropsychiatric HIV Rating Scale (NARS). The Physical Self Maintenance Scale (PSMS; Lawton & Brody, 1969) is a widely validated measure with high reliability which assesses self-care ability in six areas: toileting, feeding, dressing, grooming, ambulating, and bathing (Cronbach's alpha reliability coefficient = 0.67). The Instrumental Activities of Daily Living Scale (IADL; Lawton & Brody, 1969), an 8-item scale, measures ability in relation to telephoning, shopping, food preparation, housekeeping, laundering, use of transportation, use of medicine, and financial matters (Cronbach's alpha reliability coefficient = 0.80). In terms of validity, both the PSMS and IADL scales have been found to be highly correlated with other measures of functional and instrumental health and behavioral and adjustment ratings (Lawton & Brody, 1969). The Neuropsychiatric HIV Rating Scale (NARS; Boccellari & Dilley, 1992) is a widely used standardized measure that taps patient functional status across six cognitive and behavioral dimensions. The measure has high reliability and validity (inter-rater reliability is 95% to 96%). Construct validity of the scale has been established and it has been found to be an effective tool at correctly classifying HIV/AIDS patients with various cognitive and behavioral problems (Cronbach's alpha reliability coefficient = 0.77) (Boccellari & Dilley, 1992).

Hours of caregiving assistance provided was measured through the total number of hours of informal caregiving assistance provided per week. In addition, caregivers were asked what type of assistance they provided such as cooking, transportation, bathing feeding, toileting, administering medications, and coordinating care (Fredriksen-Goldsen & Scharlach, 2001). *Caregiver health status* was measured by a widely used single-item, 1 = poor to 4 = excellent (Maddox & Douglass, 1973). *Caregiving strain* was based on four questions regarding the degree of physical, financial or emotional and overall strain caregivers experienced due to their caregiving responsibilities. The items were scored on a four-point Likert scale (1 = none at all to 4 = a great deal). The mean was obtained for the 4 items (Cronbach's alpha reliability coefficient = 0.85) (Fredriksen-Goldsen & Scharlach, 2001). Conflict was measured through 7 items that assessed the degree of conflict in the caregiver's social network and the mean was obtained for the 7 items (Cronbach's alpha reliability coefficient = 0.71) (O'Brien, Wortman, Kessler & Joseph, 1993). *Multiple loss* experienced by caregivers was measured through a single-item asking how many people the caregiver had lost through death in the previous five years and the total number was summed. Based on questions from the National Work Study questionnaire, *discrimination* was measured by two questions regarding how often the respondent felt discriminated against on the basis of HIV/AIDS and sexual orientation. The questions were scored on a four-point Likert scale and mean was obtained for the two items (1 = rarely or none of the time to 4 = most or all of the time).

Protective factors: Caregiver optimism was assessed using the Revised Life Orientation Test (LOT-R), a 10 item measure examining the extent to which respondents are optimistic about their futures and expect the best in times of uncertainty (4-point Likert scale, strongly agreed to strongly disagree) (Carver, 1985) (Cronbach's alpha reliability coefficient = 0.70). A six-item *empowerment* scale was constructed by adapting an earlier empowerment measure (Gutierrez, Oh, & Gilmore, 2000) to insure relevance for caregivers of people with HIV/AIDS. The measure included questions regarding the extent to respondents felt able to accomplish their personal goals, lived according to their own personal values, and felt strong and capable (Cronbach's alpha reliability coefficient = 0.64). *Spiritual orientation* was based upon 3-items assessing the extent to which respondents found new faith, discovered what was important in life and prayed as a result of the difficulties in their lives (Cronbach's alpha reliability coefficient = 0.68). Caregiver *informal social support* was measured by the perceived availability of support through 7 items regarding the availability of someone if the respondent was upset and wanted to talk, had an important personal problem, needed someone to provide care if confined to a bed, needed to borrow money or get a ride to the doctor, needed guidance or needed advice in making a decision (Cronbach's alpha reliability coefficient = 0.85) (O'Brien, Wortman, Kessler & Joseph, 1993).

Outcome measures: Psychological well-being was measured by the Index of Well-Being Scale (IWB) (Campbell et al., 1976). This scale consists of two parts, general affect and life satisfaction, measured by 9 items on a 7-point Likert scale (Cronbach's alpha reliability coefficient = 0.69). *Caregiving distress* experienced by the caregiver was assessed by asking respondents to rate separately the extent to which they currently experienced physical, financial, or emotional strain as a result of their family-care responsibilities. The items were scored on a four-point Likert Scale (1 = none at all to 4 = a great deal). The Cronbach's alpha reliability coefficient = 0.89.

Data Analysis

In order to examine the relationship between the variables in the study, several methods were utilized. First, distributions on all variables were examined to identify statistical outliers and to help inform scaling decisions and the choice of analytic techniques. Proportions (if indicated), means, and standard deviations were computed for each variable. Descriptive statistics for the outcome variables and other explanatory factors are provided in Table 1.

As part of the multivariate analysis, all bivariate relationships were assessed for multicollinearity. Separate analyses were performed for the two outcome variables: psychological well-being and distress. Step-wise multiple regression models were estimated to examine the impact of background characteristics and risk and protective factors in relation to each of the outcome variables. Background characteristics were entered first followed by risk and protective factors. For the purposes of the regressions, dummy variables were created for gender (0 = female, 1 = male) and ethnicity (0 = White, 1 = Nonwhite), and the remaining variables were treated as continuous. In this paper only the data obtained from the caregivers were included in the analyses.

FINDINGS

Background Characteristics

The caregivers ranged in age from 19-74 years old, with an average age of 43 years. Sixty-nine percent of the caregivers were Caucasian, 9% African American, 7% Hispanic, 5% Asian or Pacific Islander, 1% Native American, 3% other, and 6% of mixed race. Nearly four-fifths of

TABLE 1. Descriptive Statistics for Caregiver Psychological Well-Being and Distress, and Selected Explanatory Factors

Variables	Mean	SD	Range	Cronbach Alpha Reliability Coefficient
Outcomes				
Well-being	6.51	1.93	.50-10.00	.69
Distress	1.84	.63	0.00-4.00	.89
Risk factors				
CR ADL	2.57	.29	1.85-3.26	.67
CR IADL	.37	.42	0.00-2.00	.80
CR Cognitive Impairment	.73	.74	0.00-2.67	.77
CG Health Status	2.07	.56	1.17-4.00	.64
Hours of Care	4.85	1.58	2.00-7.00	NA
CG strain	2.16	.75	0.00-4.00	.85
Conflict	2.72	.90	1.00-5.00	.71
Discrimination	1.66	.53	1.00-3.00	NA
Multiple Loss	7.46	14.48	0-150	NA
Protective factors				
Optimism	2.53	.31	1.83-4.00	.70
Spirituality	1.47	.86	0.00-3.00	.68
Empowerment	3.02	.42	2.17-4.00	.64
Social Support	4.17	.78	1.57-5.00	.85

the caregivers were male (79%) and one-fifth were female. Eighty-two percent of the caregivers self-identified as gay or lesbian.

The caregivers were most likely to have household incomes under $20,000 (39%), followed by 31% with incomes between $20,000-$39,999. Three percent had not completed high school, 19% had a high school diploma, 45% had some college and 33% had a college or advanced degree. Fifty-four percent of the informal caregivers were currently employed. More than half of the caregivers (59%) were married or partnered.

Caregiving Responsibilities

Examples of the types of caregiving assistance provided included running errands, housekeeping, cooking (more than three-quarters); assisting with home maintenance, transportation, providing financial support (more than 50%); and, personal care such as assisting with eating, bathing and administering medications (one-fifth). Over ninety percent were providing emotional support and 35% were arranging outside help. Twenty-one percent of the informal caregivers were providing 2 to 3 hours of assistance, 19% were providing 5-9 hours, 28% were providing 10-19 hours, and 32% were providing 20 or more hours of care per week.

When asked to indicate their relationship to the care recipient, 42% indicated it was their partner or spouse, 40% friend, 10% biological family member (such as parent, child or other relative), and 8% were neighbors or some other relationship. Four-fifths of the caregivers in this study were primary caregivers, with 34% being the only informal caregiver providing assistance. More than 60% said it would be helpful to receive more assistance with their care responsibilities.

The majority of caregivers in this study were caring for moderately impaired care recipients, with more than 70% of the care recipients having been hospitalized due to an HIV-related condition. In terms of multiple loss, during the past 5 years, 25% of the caregivers had lost one person through death, 36% had lost 2-5 persons, 17% 5-9 persons, and 22% had lost 10 or more persons.

Caregiving responsibilities impacted the physical, financial and emotional well-being of the majority of the caregivers. Physical strain due to caregiving was reported by 64% of the caregivers; emotional strain was reported by 86% and financial strain by 58%. Despite the difficulties they faced in their lives, more than 70% of the caregivers were moderately to highly satisfied with their lives. Thirty-three percent of the caregivers caring for persons with high levels of disability and poor health reported high levels of psychological well-being.

Predictors of Distress and Well-Being

Step-wise multiple regression analyses were performed to examine the contribution to the outcome variables self-reported by caregiver of well-being and distress made by the background characteristics and risk and protective factors, as shown in Table 2. Background characteristics entered into the regression for psychological well-being and distress included age, income, race, gender, and education. Risk factors included the health status and ADL/IADL and cognitive impairment levels of the persons with HIV/AIDS, health status of the caregiver, hours of assistance provided, caregiver strain, conflict, discrimination, and multiple loss. Protective factors entered into the model included optimism, spiritual orientation, self-empowerment, and social support.

TABLE 2. Stepwise Multiple Regressions of Caregiver Well-Being and Distress, on Demographic and Background Characteristics, and Risk and Protective Factors (Standardized Betas)

Factor	Well-being	Distress
Background characteristics		
Gender	.07	−.13*
Ethnicity	.13	.07
Age	.01	.04
Education	−.03	.04
Income	.17*	−.03
R	.02	.01
Risk factors		
CR ADL	.10	.20**
CR IADL	−.01	.19**
CR Cognitive Impairment	.04	−.11
CG Health Status	−.35***	.06
Hours of Assistance	−.11	.16*
Caregiving Strain	−.12	.46***
Conflict	.01	.08
Discrimination	−.17*	.09
Multiple Loss	−.17*	.01
R²	.26	.47
Protective factors		
CG Optimism	.15*	.02
Spiritual Orientation	−.09	−.06
Empowerment	.21*	−.16*
Social Support	.08	−.11
R²	.32	.50
R² (Total)	.32	.50

* p < .05
** p < .01
*** p < .001

The model predicted 50% of the variance in caregiver distress. Significant predictors of distress included being female, higher levels of ADL/IADL impairment in the care recipient, higher levels of strain experienced by the caregiver, providing more hours of assistance, and lower levels of caregiver empowerment. The model predicted 32% of the variance in psychological well-being. Factors that contributed significantly to well-being included higher income, greater caregiver health, higher levels of caregiver optimism and self-empowerment, and lower levels of discrimination and multiple loss.

DISCUSSION

This study provides important new information concerning several understudied aspects of HIV/AIDS caregiving including more fully understanding the variations in outcomes, as well as the differing types of risk and protective factors that are salient in predicting distress and well-being. In this study there was high variation in caregiving outcomes with many caregivers demonstrating high levels of psychological well-being despite adverse life circumstances such as the poor health of the person living with HIV/AIDS.

Traditional stress and coping paradigms have long dominated caregiving research, highlighting the extent of distress associated with caregiving. The levels of caregiver distress in this study and its predictors mirror those found in previous caregiving research, with significant factors including the characteristics of the caregiver, care recipient, and the caregiving situation, such as the patient's health status and functional impairment (Irving et al., 1995; Siegel, Ravies & Krauss, 1991) and the extent of care provided (Miller & Montgomery, 1987).

Overall, the majority of caregiving studies in the general caregiving literature suggest that informal care for a relative with disabilities results in negative consequences for the caregiver and their families (Owens, 2001; Polen & Green, 2001). Caregiving is repeatedly associated with decreased psychological health among caregivers, including increased levels of caregiver burden, role strain and depression (Polen & Green, 2001; Berg-Weger, Rubio & Tebb, 2000; Hans & Haley, 1999).

Although HIV/AIDS caregiving has repeatedly been found to be associated with increased levels of distress (Callery, 2000; Turner & Catania, 1997; Wight, 2000, 2002; Wight, LeBlanc & Aneshenesel, 1998), less is known about caregiver well-being. As noted earlier, caregiver well-being is most often operationalized as lower levels or the absence of distress (Yates, Tennstedt & Bei-Hung Chang, 1999; George & Gwyther, 1986). The limited conceptual clarification between caregiver distress and well-being hinders the understanding of antecedents that lead to caregiver well-being and other positive outcomes. In this study differing types of antecedents were predictive of distress and well-being, suggesting that the two concepts need to be treated as conceptually distinct.

Caregiver income and health status, discrimination, multiple loss, dispositional optimism, and empowerment emerged as significant variables predicting well-being in this study.

Many of these factors have been largely neglected in the general caregiving research yet they may be particularly salient within historically disadvantaged communities. For example, caregivers with lower incomes and poor health have been found to experience higher care demands and to have fewer resources to meet their caregiving responsibilities (Fredriksen-Goldsen & Scharlach, 2001). Because of their history of marginalization and invisibility, lesbians and gay men may encounter specific obstacles in receiving and providing care, such as multiple loss, discrimination in health and long-term care settings, limited access to formal service, and lack of legal protection for their loved ones.

Many of the caregivers in this study experienced high levels of loss due to death, which was associated with lower levels of well-being. The rate of HIV/AIDS related deaths has been catastrophic in the gay and lesbian community. Many of these losses have been nonnormative in terms of age given that the disease has affected many persons with HIV/AIDS and their caregivers early in life. While rituals have been established in the gay community as a result of the HIV/AIDS epidemic, many still perceive a lack of support for grief and bereavement in the community (Richard, Wrubel, & Folkman, 2000; Simmons, 1999).

Despite more than twenty years of HIV/AIDS-related public health education, HIV/AIDS continues to be a stigmatizing health condition, and discrimination against people with HIV/AIDS continues. In one survey nearly 20% (18.7%) of the respondents agreed with the following statement: "People who get AIDS through sex or drug use have gotten what they deserve." One fourth also reported misinformed opinions on HIV transmission (Centers for Disease Control and Preventions, 2002b). Many HIV-related caregivers report feeling discouraged by the level of discrimination they encounter (Poindexter, 2001), and it is an important factor that must be considered as it impacts their well-being and overall caregiving experience.

Both optimism and empowerment emerge as significant protective factors positively associated with caregiver well-being. Optimism and self-empowerment may play important roles in how positive meaning is created through the caregiving experience (Land & Long, 2000), as well as how caregivers balance the costs of providing care with personal rewards. Among African Americans caring for family members living with HIV/AIDS many reported they were empowered to actively fight against HIV/AIDS as a result of their caregiving responsibilities

(Tolliver, 2001). In their fight against HIV/AIDS, they learned to resist stigma associated with HIV/AIDS and not accept images that marginalized them or negated what was happening to their family members (Boyle, Hodnicki & Ferrell, 1999).

The majority of caregivers in this study were gay men and lesbians providing care to partners and friends. It has been suggested that partners and friends are more likely than biological family members to provide care due to the stigmatized nature of HIV/AIDS (Kadushin, 1996) and the informal extended family networks that exist within the gay and lesbian community (Fredriksen-Goldsen, 2003). It continues to be important to use a broad definition of family that is based on commitment when developing interventions and policies to support caregivers and those living with HIV/AIDS.

In this study, men far outnumbered women as caregivers, a finding consistent with HIV/AIDS care, but inconsistent with the general caregiving literature as well the popular notion that women have primary caregiving responsibilities. Similar to the findings in the general caregiving literature, being female in this study was associated with higher levels of distress. While the experiences of male caregivers have largely gone unrecognized in caregiving services and research, male caregivers have reported difficulty in being recognized as caregivers and acquiring support for their care responsibilities (Kramer & Thompson, 2002). Given the high prevalence of male caregivers and the extent of care being provided within the context of same sex couples, HIV/AIDS care provides a unique opportunity to further explore differences in the care experience as they intersect with both gender and gender roles.

There continues to be a need for interventions designed to assist family members caring for those living with HIV/AIDS (Stajduhar & Davies, 1998). The findings from this study suggest that rather than solely organize caregiving interventions toward the reduction of distress, it may be important to tailor such programs to increase caregiver well-being as well. Interventions aimed at nurturing optimism among informal caregivers, designing methods to empower them to resist the stigma they face as well as finding new ways to be responsive to the discrimination and multiple losses they encounter may provide important tools for increasing caregiver well-being. Helping caregivers find a balance between the role that HIV/AIDS plays in their own personal lives as well as getting involved in HIV related issues outside of the immediate caregiving situation may foster a personal sense of empowerment and help establish a larger meaning to the caregiving experience (Carlisle, 2000). Treating caregiving as a multidimensional construct that includes both positive and negative outcomes is critical to developing interventions that seek to decrease risk and increase their capacities as caregivers.

Contrary to the findings in the general caregiving literature (Chang, Noonan, Tennstedt, 1998; Kelly et al., 1993; Lackner et al., 1993; Magana, 1999; Shafran, 2001; Tolliver, 2001), religious orientation and social support were not associated with caregiver distress or well-being in this study. Items utilized to measure religious or spiritual orientation constructs may need to be modified to increase their applicability to these caregivers given the history of marginalization within many religious and faith communities. Furthermore, the variation in social support among these caregivers may be limited given the extent of death and loss experienced by the majority of them. Additional measures of both spirituality and social support need to be further examined to assess their role within these communities.

While the findings from this study suggest that well-being and distress are conceptually distinct, more research with larger sample sizes is needed to further explore and model the relationship between distress and well-being as well as the role of risk and protective factors. This study is exploratory in nature and the findings are not necessarily reflective of caregivers in general, nor can the findings be generalized beyond the specific sample. While the resilience model used in this research more clearly addresses caregiver well-being than has previous HIV/AIDS studies, it does not account for a substantial portion of the variance in the outcome variables. Additional research is needed to examine and specify the components of well-being as well as to explore the impact of additional individual, cultural and community-level variables that may serve a protective function for caregivers assisting gay men with HIV/AIDS. Longitudinal studies are also necessary to begin examining resilience as a developmental process as well as to explore the impact of caregiving over the life course.

CONCLUSION

HIV/AIDS continues to be a serious public health issue, and the findings from this study indicate that caregiving entails more than distress and that future research needs to consider the well-being and resilience of informal caregivers. Our understanding of the caregiving process is enhanced by treating caregiving as a multidimensional construct that includes both positive and negative outcomes. Studying an historically disadvantaged group, such as gay men living with HIV/AIDS and their caregivers, can expand our knowledge about the diversity of caregiving needs and types of effective supports. The development of a community-based system of care depends on finding effective ways to help caregivers confront the adversity they face, and supporting and enhancing their strengths. The resilience of caregivers needs to be recognized and integrated into the design of innovative, culturally appropriate interventions that support both informal caregivers and persons living with HIV/AIDS.

REFERENCES

Aneshensel, C. S., Pearlin, L. I., Mullan, J. R., Zarit, S. H., and Whitlatch, C. J. (1995). *Profiles in caregiving: The unexpected career.* New York: Academic Press.

Boccellari, A. A., & Dilley, J. W. (1992). Management and residential placement problems of patients with HIV-related cognitive impairment. *Hospital and Community Psychiatry, 43*(1), 32-37.

Boyle, J. S., Hodnicki, D. R., & Ferrell, J. A. (1999). Patterns of resistance: African American mothers and adult children with HIV illness. *Scholarly Inquiry for Nursing Practice, 13*(2), 111-133.

Bunting, S. M. (2001). Sustaining the relationship: Women's caregiving in the context of HIV disease. *Health Care for Women International, 22*(1-2), 131-148.

Burggraf, V. (1999). *Burden, depression, physical health status, social support, and absenteeism: A study of employed and unemployed caregivers of the elderly.* Unpublished dissertation.

Callery, K. E. (2000). *The role of stigma and psycho-social factors on perceived caregiver burden in HIV/AIDS gay male caregivers.* Unpublished dissertation.

Campbell, A., Converse, P. E., & Rogers, W. L. (1976). *The quality of American life: Perceptions, evaluations and satisfaction. Index of Well-Being Scale (IWB).* New York: Sage.

Carlisle, C. (2000). The search for meaning in HIV and AIDS: The carers' experience. *Qualitative Health Research, 10*(6), 750-765.

Center for Disease Control. (2002a). Update: AIDS–United States, 2000. *Morbidity and Mortality Weekly Report, 51*(27), 592-595.

Center for Disease Control. (2002b). Notice to Readers: World AIDS Day, December 1, 2002. *Morbidity and Mortality Weekly Report, 51*(47), 1074-1075.

Centers for Disease Control and Prevention (2003). *HIV/AIDS Surveillance Report 2002. 14,* 1-40.

Chang, B. H., Noonan, A. E., & Tennstedt, S. L. (1998). The role of religion/spirituality in coping with caregiving for disabled elders. *Gerontologist, 38*(4), 463-470.

Chang, B. L., Becht, M.L., & Carter, P.A. (2001). Predictors of social support and caregiver outcomes. *Women & Health, 33*(1-2), 39-61.

Chappell, N. L., & Reid, R. C. (2002). Burden and well-being among caregivers: Examining the distinction. *The Gerontologist, 42*(6), 772-780.

Clipp, E. C., Adinolfi, A. J., Forrest, L., & Bennett, C. L. (1995). Informal caregivers of persons with AIDS. *Journal of Palliative Care, 11*(2), 10-18.

Cowles, K. V., & Rodgers, B. L. (1994). Significant others of persons with AIDS: A preliminary study. *Journal of Gay and Lesbian Psychotherapy, 2*(2), 101-119.

Folkman, S., Chesney, M.A., & Christopher-Richards, A. (1994). Stress and coping in caregiving partners of men with AIDS. *Psychiatric Clinics of North America, 17*(1), 35-53.

Folkman, S., Chesney, M. A., Cooke, M., Boccellari, A. A., & Collette, L. (1994). Caregiver burden in HIV-positive and HIV-negative partners of men with AIDS. *Journal of Consulting and Clinical Psychology, 62*(4), 746-756.

Fredriksen, K. I. (1993). *The provision of informal adult care: The impact of family and employment responsibilities.* Unpublished Dissertation, University of California, Berkeley, CA.

Fredriksen, K. I. (1996). Gender differences in employment and the informal care of adults. *Journal of Women & Aging, 8*(2), 35-53.

Fredriksen, K. I., & Farwell, N. (In press). Dual responsibilities of family care and employment among Black, Hispanic, Asian and White caregivers: Implications for social work practice. *Gerontological Social Work.*

Fredriksen-Goldsen, K., & Scharlach, A. E. (2001). *Families and work: New directions in the twenty-first century.* New York: Oxford University Press.

Fredriksen-Goldsen, K. (2003). *Multigenerational Health and AIDS Caregiving.* Paper presented at the Council of Social Work Annual Meeting, Atlanta, Georgia.

Garcia, E. (2000). Caregiving in the context of ethnicity: Hispanic caregiver wives of stroke patients. Unpublished Dissertation.

Garwick, A. W., Kohrman, C. H., Titus, J. C., Wolman, C., & Blum, R. (1999). Variations in families' explanations of childhood chronic conditions: A cross-cultural perspective. In H. I. McCubbin & A. I. Thompson (Eds.), *The dynamics of resilient families* (Vol. 4). Thousand Oaks, CA: Sage.

George, L. K., & Gwyther, L. P. (1986). Caregiver well-being: A multidimensional examination of family caregivers of demented adults. *The Gerontologist, 26*(3), 253-259.

Gerstel, N., & Gallagher, S. K. (1993). Kinkeeping and distress: Gender, recipients of care, and work-family conflict. *Journal of Marriage and the Family, 55*(3), 598-608.

Gove, P. B. (1993). Webster's Third New International Dictionary. Springfield, MA: Merriam-Webster, Inc.

Gutierrez, L., Oh, H. J., & Gillmore, M. R. (2000). Toward an understanding of (Em)Power(Ment) for HIV/AIDS prevention with adolescent women. *Sex Roles, 42*, 581-611.

Harwood, D. G., Barker, W. W., Ownby, R. L, Bravo, M, Agueroa, H, Duara, R. (2000). Predictors of positive and negative appraisal among Cuban American caregivers of Alzheimer's disease patients. *International Journal of Geriatric Psychiatry, 15*(6), 481-487.

Irving, G., Bor, R., & Catalan, J. (1995). Psychological distress among gay men supporting a lover or partner with AIDS: A pilot study. *AIDS Care, 7*(5), 605-617.

Kadushin, G. (1996). Gay men with AIDS and their families of origin: An analysis of social support. *Health and Social Work, 21*(2), 141-147.

Kelly, J. A., Murphy, D. A., Bahr, G. R., Koob, J. J., Morgan, M. G., Kalichman, S. C., et al. (1993). Factors associated with severity of depression and high risk sexual behavior among persons diagnosed with Human Immunodeficiency Virus (HIV) infection. *Health Psychology, 12*(3), 215-219.

Kramer, B. J., & Kipnis, S. (1995). Eldercare and work-role conflict: Toward an understanding of gender differences in caregiver burden. *Gerontologist, 35*(3), 340-348.

Kramer, B. J., & Thompson, E. H. (Eds.). (2002). *Men as caregivers: Theory, research, and service implications.* New York: Springer Publishing.

Lackner, J. B., Joseph, J. G., Ostrow, D. G., & Eshleman, S. (1993). The effects of social support on Hopkins Symptom Checklist-assessed depression and distress in a cohort of Human Immunodeficiency Virus-positive and -negative gay men. *Journal of Nervous and Mental Disease, 181*(10), 632-638.

Land, H., & Long, J. D. (2000). The structure of coping in AIDS caregivers: A factor analytically derived measure. *Journal of Applied Social Psychology, 30*(3), 463-483.

Lawton, M. P., & Brody, E. M. (1969). Assessment of older people: Self-maintaining and instrumental activities of daily living. *Gerontologist, 7,* 179-186.

LeBlanc, A. J., Aneshensel, C. S., & Wright, R. G. (1995). Psychotherapy use and depression among AIDS caregivers. *Journal of Community Psychology, 23,* 127-142.

Maddox, G.L., & Douglass, E.B. (1973). Self-assessment of health: A longitudinal study of elderly subjects. *Journal of Health and Social Behavior, 14:*87-93.

Magana, S. M. (1999). Puerto Rican families caring for an adult with mental retardation: Role of familism. *American Journal on Mental Retardation, 104*(5), 466.

Majerovitz, D. (2001). Formal versus informal support: Stress buffering among dementia caregivers. *Journal of Mental Health and Aging, 7*(4), 413-423.

McCubbin, M., & McCubbin, H. I. (1993). Family coping with health crises: The resiliency model of family stress, adjustment and adaptation. In C. Danielson, B. Hamel-Bissell & P. Winstead-Fry (Eds.), *Families health and illness.* New York: Mosby.

Miller, B., & Montgomery, A. (1987). *Developing a measurement model of spousal caregiver strain, stress and satisfaction.* Paper presented at the Annual Meeting of the Gerontological Society of America, Washington, DC.

Miller, B., Townsend, A., Carpenter, E., Montgomery, R., Stull, D., & Young, R. (2001). Social support and caregiver distress: A replication analysis. *Journals of Gerontology: Series B: Psychological Sciences and Social Sciences, 56B*(4), S249-S256.

Mullan, J. T. (1998). Aging and informal caregiving to people with HIV/AIDS. *Research on Aging, 20*(6), 712-738.

Nimmons, D. (2002). Communities of caring. In D. Nimmons (Ed.), *The soul beneath the skin: The unseen hearts and habits of gay men,* (pp. 40-55). New York: St. Martin's Press.

O'Brien, K., Wortman, -. C. B., Kessler, R. C., & Joseph, J. G. (1993). Social relationships of men at risk for AIDS. *Social Science and Medicine, 36*(9), 1161-1167.

Ory, M. G., and Hoffman, R. R. III, Yee, J. L., Tennstedt, S., and Schulz, R. (1999). Prevalence and impact of caregiving: A detailed comparison between dementia and non-dementia caregivers. *The Gerontologist, 39,* 177-185.

Owens, S. D. (2001). African American female elder caregivers: An analysis of the Psychosocial correlates of their stress level, alcohol use and psychological well-being. Unpublished Dissertation.

Pearlin, L. I., Mullan, J. T., Semple, S. J., and Skaff, M. M. (1990). Caregiving and the stress process: An overview of concepts and their measures. *The Gerontologist, 30*(5), 583-591.

Pearlin, L. I., Mullan, J. T., Aneshensel, C. S., Wadlaw, L., & Harrington, C. (1994). The structure and functions of AIDS caregiving relationships. *Psychosocial Rehabilitation Journal, 17*(4), 52-67.

Poindexter, C. I. (2001). "I'm still blessed." The assets and needs of HIV-affected caregivers over 50. *Families in Society, 82*(5), 525-536.

Radloff, L. (1977). The CES-D Scale: A self-report depression scale for research in the general population. *Applied Psychological Measurement, 1*(3), 385-401.

Rait, D. S. (1991). The family context of AIDS. *Psychiatric Medicine, 9,* 423-439.

Raveis, V. H., & Siegel, K. (1991, February). The impact of caregiving on informal of familial care givers. *AIDS Patient Care,* 39-43.

Richards, T. A., Acree, M., & Folkman, S. (1999). Spiritual aspects of loss among partners of men with AIDS: Postbereavement follow-up. *Death Studies, 23*(2), 105-127.

Richards, T. A., Wrubel, J., & Folkman, S. (2000). Death rites in the San Francisco gay community: Cultural developments of the AIDS epidemic. *Omega: Journal of Death and Dying, 40*(2), 335-350.

Robinson, D. L. (1997). Family stress theory: Implications for family health. *Journal of the American Academy of Nurse Practitioners, 9*(1), 17-23.

Rungreangkulkij, S. (2000). Experience of Thai families of a person with schizophrenia: Family stress and adaptation. *Dissertation-Abstracts-International:-Section-B:-The-Sciences-and-Engineering, 61*(8-B), 4080.

Scharlach, A. E., & Fredriksen, K. I. (1994). Elder care versus adult care: Does care recipient age make a difference? *Research on Aging, 16,* 43-68.

Shafran, R. D. (2001). The role of religion in coping with caring for an adult family member with severe and persistent mental illness. Unpublished Dissertation.

Siegel, K., Raveis, V. H., & Kraus, D. (1994). Psychological well-being of gay men with AIDS: Contribution of positive and negative illness-related network interactions to depressive mood. *Social Science and Medicine, 39,* 11.

Simmons, L. E. (1999). *The grief experience of HIV-positive gay men who lose partners to AIDS.* Unpublished dissertation.

Sipes, C. S. (1998). *The experiences of gay male caregivers who provided care for their partners with AIDS.* Unpublished dissertation.

Sipes, C. S. (2002). The experiences and relationships of gay male caregivers who provide care for their partners with AIDS. In B. J. Kramer & E. H. Thompson (Eds.), *Men as caregivers: Theory, research, and service implications* (pp. 151-189). New York: Springer Publishing.

Soskolne, V., Acree, M., & Folkman, S. (2000). Social support and mood in gay caregivers of men with AIDS. *AIDS and Behavior, 4*(3), 221-232.

Stajduhar, K. I., & Davies, B. (1998). Palliative care at home: Reflections on HIV/AIDS family caregiving experiences. *Journal of Palliative Care, 14*(2), 14-22.

Stewart, A. L., Hays, R. D., & Ware, J. E. (1988). The MOS Short-form General Heath Survey. *Medical Care, 26*(7), 724-735.

Svavarsdottir, E., McCubbin, M., & Kane, J. (2000). Well-being of parents of young children with asthma. *Research in Nursing and Health, 23,* 346-358.

Tolliver, D. E. (2001). African American female caregivers of family members living with HIV/AIDS. *Families in Society, 82*(2), 145-156.

Turner, H. A., Catania, J. A., & Gagnon, J. (1994). The prevalence of informal caregiving to persons with AIDS in the United States: Caregiver characteristics and their implications. *Social Science and Medicine, 38*(11), 1543-1552.

Turner, H. A., & Catania, J. A. (1997). Informal caregiving to persons with AIDS in the United States: Caregiver burden among central cities residents eighteen to forty-nine years old. *American Journal of Community Psychology, 25*(1), 35-59.

Turner, H. A., Pearlin, L. I., & Mullan, J. T. (1998). Sources and determinants of social support for caregivers of persons with AIDS. *Journal of Health and Social Behavior, 39*(2), 137-151.

UNAIDS, (2004, June). *2004 Report on the global AIDS epidemic: Executive Summary* [English Original], 1-18. The Joint United Nations Programme on HIV/AIDS: Geneva, Switzerland.

Walsh, F. (2002). A family resilience framework: Innovative practice applications. *Family Relations, 51*(2), 130-137.

Walsh, F. (1998). Foundations of a family resilience approach. In F. Walsh (Ed.) *Strengthening family resilience*, (pp. 3-25). New York: Guilford Press.

Walsh, F. (1996). The concept of family resilience: Crisis and challenge. *Family Process, 35*(3), 261-281.

Wight, R. G., LeBlanc, A. J., & Aneshensel, C. S. (1998). AIDS caregiving and health among midlife and older women. *Health Psychology, 17*(2), 130-137.

Wight, R. G. (2000). Precursive depression among HIV infected AIDS caregivers over time. *Social Science and Medicine, 51*(5), 759-770.

Wight, R. G. (2002). AIDS caregiving stress among HIV-infected men. In B. J. Kramer & E. H. Thompson (Eds.), *Men as caregivers: Theory, research, and service implications* (pp. 190-212). New York: Springer Publishing.

World Health Organization. (2002). *AIDS Epidemic Update 2002.*

Zak, M. (2000). The impact of post-stroke aphasia and accompanying neuropsychological deficits on caregiving spouses and marriage. Unpublished Dissertation.

doi:10.1300/J041v18n03_04

Caregiving Experiences Among American Indian Two-Spirit Men and Women: Contemporary and Historical Roles

Teresa Evans-Campbell
Karen I. Fredriksen-Goldsen
Karina L. Walters
Antony Stately

SUMMARY. Many Native men and women embrace the term *two-spirit* to capture their sexuality and gender expression. By analyzing the narratives of almost 70 two-spirit Native leaders from across the U.S., we explored contemporary experiences of caregiving among two-spirit people, historical two-spirit roles related to caregiving, and the implications of these roles for two-spirit and Native communities. The central role of

Teresa Evans-Campbell, PhD, is Assistant Professor and Director of the Institute for Indigenous Health and Child Welfare Research, School of Social Work, University of Washington, 4101 15th Ave. NE, Seattle, WA 98105 (E-mail: tecamp@u.washington.edu).

Karen I. Fredriksen-Goldsen, PhD, is Associate Professor and Director, Institute for Multigenerational Health, School of Social Work, University of Washington, Seattle, WA.

Karina L. Walters, PhD, is Associate Professor, School of Social Work, and Director of the Institute for Indigenous Wellness Research at the University of Washington.

Antony Stately, PhD, is Project Director of the HONOR Project, School of Social Work, University of Washington.

[Haworth co-indexing entry note]: "Caregiving Experiences Among American Indian Two-Spirit Men and Women: Contemporary and Historical Roles." Evans-Campbell, Teresa et al. Co-published simultaneously in *Journal of Gay & Lesbian Social Services* (The Haworth Press, Inc.) Vol. 18, No. 3/4, 2007, pp. 75-92; and: *Caregiving with Pride* (ed: Karen I. Fredriksen-Goldsen) The Haworth Press, Inc., 2007, pp. 75-92. Single or multiple copies of this article are available for a fee from The Haworth Document Delivery Service [1-800-HAWORTH, 9:00 a.m. - 5:00 p.m. (EST). E-mail address: docdelivery@haworthpress.com].

caregiving among two-spirit people, related Native community expectations, the diversity of caregiving experiences across the lifespan, and the importance of caregiving in maintaining indigenous community ties emerged as key themes. doi:10.1300/J041v18n03_05 *[Article copies available for a fee from The Haworth Document Delivery Service: 1-800-HAWORTH. E-mail address: <docdelivery@haworthpress.com> Website: <http://www. HaworthPress.com> © 2007 by The Haworth Press, Inc. All rights reserved.]*

KEYWORDS. American Indian/Alaskan Native, GLBT spirituality, GLBT men and women of color, two-spirit, sexual orientation and discrimination, caregiving, parenting, qualitative research

INTRODUCTION

To date relatively little is known about caregiving in racial and ethnic minority communities. Importantly, the limited scholarship available has identified ethnic and racial differences in caregiving values and norms (Dilworth-Anderson, Williams, & Gibson, 2002; Foley, Tung, & Mutran, 2002), informal social support networks (Ortiz, Simmons, & Hinton, 1999), access to caregiving services (Talamantes, Lawler, & Espino, 1995), and service utilization (Hinrichsen & Ramirez, 1992; Thornton, 1998). When controlling for the disability level of the care recipient, for example, ethnic minority caregivers tend to provide assistance for longer periods of time and use fewer formal supports than White caregivers (Dilworth-Andersen, Williams & Cooper, 1999; Fredriksen-Goldsen & Farwell, 2004; McCann, Hebert, Beckett, Morris, Scherr, & Evans, 2000; Peek, Coward, & Peek, 2000). Notably, the majority of existing studies compare the experiences of African American and White caregivers of elders (Fredman et al., 1995; Gitlin, et. al., 2001; Martin, 2000; Young & Kahana, 1995), and we know much less about the experiences and needs of American Indian/Alaska Native (hereafter referred to as Native) caregivers.

Studies examining informal caregiving in Native communities have focused primarily on the care of elders and factors associated with caregiver burden. Caregiver burden in Native communities has been described as multidimensional, incorporating role conflict, negative feelings, guilt and caregiver efficacy (John, Hennessey, Dyeson, & Garrett, 2001). Numerous factors related to Native caregiver burden have been identified and include: (1) distress and anxiety related to managing in-home medical care, (2) difficulties with psychosocial aspects of care, (3) stress on family relationships, and (4) negative impacts on the caregiver's health and well-being (Hennessey & John, 1996). Hennessey and John (1995) found that many Native American caregivers respond to such demands by expanding their social support network and securing additional caregiving resources. It is also important to note that Native people tend to develop chronic health conditions at younger ages compared to those from other ethnic groups (Hennessey, John, & Anderson, 1999; Jervis & Manson, 2002) and, as a consequence, Native people may be more likely to serve as caregivers, they may provide care for relatively longer periods of time, and they may provide care for others while experiencing their own health concerns.

Although preliminary research among Native communities suggest that caregiver burden exists, there are considerable cultural differences in the expression of caregiver burden and how it is experienced in relation to cultural role expectations. Caregiving roles are valued and proscribed for individuals as they mature and reach elder status in many Native communities. In many cases, caregiving roles are not defined by illness or distress but rather by roles of nurturing and passing on of knowledge in relation to elder status. Thus, while the case of Native grandparents caring for grandchildren may be framed as a "burden" from a Western perspective, in many Native cultures intergenerational caregiving is a cultural expectation consistent with status responsibilities (familial, elder, and communal). Additionally, the challenges of Native caregiving are buffered with meaningful extended family ties and supports from significant others. As a consequence, the issue of "burden" in relation to caregiving for Native Peoples may have more to do with the level of unanticipated role stress or resource stress (e.g., lack of relatives for social support) than to the actual caregiving activity per se. An early study comparing caregiver burden among Caucasian and Native American caregivers, for example, found that Native caregivers tended to perceive less control over the care situation and were more likely to acknowledge benefits resulting from caregiving (Strong, 1984). Native caregivers may also be more likely to contextualize challenging caregiving situations within cultural norms and values. For example, in some tribes Western diagnosed dementia-related hallucinations represent an elder's contact with the spirit world and are viewed as a source of strength rather than a sign of dysfunction (Henderson & Traphagan, 2005). Finally, Native caregivers view caregiving as a collective and holistic enterprise; and, as a result, experience caregiving at multiple levels–individual, familial, communal–rather than interpreting it solely from the perspective of their own individual lives (Hennessey & John, 1995, 1996; Hennessey et al., 1999).

TWO-SPIRIT PEOPLE IN INDIGENOUS COMMUNITIES

Although many Native people serve as caregivers at some point in their lives, Native LGBTQT-S (lesbian, gay, bi-sexual, transgender, queer, or two-spirit; hereafter referred to as two-spirit) people often have specific cultural roles and responsibilities tied to caregiving in indigenous communities (Jacobs, Thomas, & Lang, 1997; Walters, Evans-Campbell, Simoni, Bhuyan, & Ronquillo, 2006). Moreover, these roles are intimately tied to their identities as Native LGBTQ or "two-spirit" people. Many indigenous societies in North America have historically acknowledged and incorporated the existence of diverse gender and sexual identities among community members (Brown, 1997; Lang, 1998; Little Crow, Wright, & Brown, 1997). Although there were exceptions, these community members tended to be well integrated within Native communities and often occupied highly respected social and ceremonial roles which included caregiving (Lang, 1998). Over the past several centuries, however, colonization has dramatically influenced the acceptance and inclusivity of those with alternative gender or sexual identities (Tinker, 1993).

While numerous scholars have explored the history and lived experience of indigenous peoples with diverse gender and sexual identities (Farrer, 1997), this work is almost exclusively focused on a bilinear Western model of gender with little or no insight into the complexity of gender identities and their intersectionality with sexual expressions. Accordingly, scholars have used limited labels such as *third gender*, *women-men*, and *men-women* (Lang, 1998) to describe Native people with multiple or alternative gender identities and/or sexual identities. Another commonly used term in gender scholarship, *berdache,* is considered offensive because of its colonial origins and purely sexual connotations: it is a non-Native term used to refer to male slaves who served as prostitutes (Jacobs, Thomas, & Lang, 1997; Thomas & Jacobs, 1999). In an attempt to capture the complex nature of indigenous gender and sexual identities, contemporary Native LGBT activists created a new term to define themselves–two-spirit. The word two-spirit derives from the Northern Algonquin word *niizh manitoag*, meaning *two-spirits*, and refers to an individual who embraces both feminine and masculine characteristics (Anguksuar, 1997). While not used by all Native LGBT people, this term is gaining acceptance and is increasingly used to define contemporary Native LGBT peoples. The term has important political and social implications for all Native people–two-spirit and other Natives–as it embraces the complexity of multi-gendered statuses and expressions, and serves to reconnect contemporary Native people with traditional conceptions of sexuality and gender identity beyond Western dualistic notions of sexual and gender expression (Walters, Evans-Campbell, Simoni, et al., 2006).

One of the primary roles discussed in scholarship related to two-spirit identity is caretaking both historically and in contemporary times. In this paper, we present findings from a large qualitative study of two-spirit people to explore experiences, perceptions, and challenges related to caregiving. The data are part of a large-scale national study of two-spirit health (i.e., the HONOR Project) conducted in seven urban sites across the country from 2004-2006.

METHODS

As part of this larger study, HONOR Project staff worked with local, national, and regional two-spirit communities and Native agencies to complete 63 in-depth interviews with two-spirit leaders covering a range of topics including identity, resilience, and caregiving. In order to identify potential interviewees, we asked HONOR Project advisory board members as well as members of two-spirit organizations to suggest the names of those they considered to be two-spirit leaders. Individuals identified as leaders were then contacted and asked to be part of the study. To be eligible, participants had to meet six criteria: (a) be American Indian, Alaskan Native, First Nations, or Metis; (b) be self-identified as LGBTQT-S; (c) be age 18 or older; (d) be English-speaking; (e) not be psychotic or demented; and (f) reside in one of the seven national urban sites included in the study.

Using participatory action research methods, study investigators developed an interview guide that incorporated nine broad questions related to two-spirit identity, social support, health, and caregiving. We used narrative and indigenist research methods in our research, allowing the two-spirit leaders to give their *testimonios*, a type of oral history and life story as two-spirit leaders (Bishop, 2005; McMahon & Rogers, 1994; Tuhiwai Smith, 2005). Participants were encouraged to tell their stories with as little interruption as possible. Interviewers did not focus on uncovering minute historical information but instead explored how historical, cultural, and social events influence two-spirit identity, roles, and wellness. Embedded in the narratives are indigenist ways of knowing, worldviews, "deep metaphors," and references to cultural traditions that connect individuals with ancestral ties as well as future generations

(Tuhiwai Smith, 2005). Participants had the option of reviewing their interview transcript and making changes if they desired.

For purposes of this paper, we conducted theoretical sampling from the qualitative interviews with 63 two-spirit activist leaders. Specifically, we read through the two-spirit interviews and selected 22 "cases" in which respondents explicitly talked about caregiving roles. As much as possible, we present the two-spirit leaders' own words to illustrate similarities and differences in how Native two-spirit people "talk" or give testimony to their caregiving experiences. All interviews were audio-taped and generally took between two and three hours.

In terms of data analytic strategies, we used a modified form of a feminist interpretive method of narrative analysis called the Listening Guide, originated by Gilligan and colleagues (Gilligan, Spencer, Weinberg, & Bertsch, 2003). Each narrative was "listened to" by reading the transcripts multiple times, by multiple readers (including a two-spirit man) with the intention of "listening" to different aspects of a particular topic (e.g., caregiving), and then re-reading the transcripts to listen or focus on a different aspect of the topic of interest each time. Sections of the transcripts were color coded creating a visual map of the narratives' layers in which identifiable, coherent "voices" could be heard. One of the authors "listened" by recording her thoughts simultaneous to color coding the transcripts, and thus, worked reflexively in interpreting the transcripts and coding the voices generating "themes" that relationally emerged across the transcripts.

The two-spirit voices reflected in these interviews represent considerable tribal, cultural, and geographic diversity. Respondents ranged in age from their early 20s through late 60s and all were considered leaders in their respective communities. To protect confidentiality, pseudonyms are used and identifying information such as tribal affiliation or site specific information about a particular community incident to which they could be linked were all deleted from their narratives. When necessary, quotes were edited to ensure readability and clarity.

RESPONSIBILITY TO THE COMMUNITY

Many of the two-spirit people we spoke with had served as caregivers at some point in their lives or anticipated taking on this role in the future. Those we interviewed often alluded to caregiving as a primary role and responsibility of a two-spirit person. Indeed, a number of respondents felt that caretaking connected them to their historical roles, at individual and community levels.

The two-spirits, we were responsible for the village. We were the ones who took care of the infirmed. We were the ones who raised the children, not because they were unwanted, or abandoned or, we were in text godparents. We were the ones who stayed behind, and protected the village; we're the last form of defense against, protecting the women, the children, and the village.

–Terri

That's what our role was in previous times [caretaking] and then so many of the people that I knew in the community . . . were kind of in a caretaking role, and then coincidentally I've met all these people who are either in the medical field or they did other things in the community to kind of bridge different parts of the communities . . . I don't think it's a coincidence that my life has gone in that direction. I dunno, I'm just really drawn to it, I really am and I felt like since I was young, you know, I always felt like for some reason I needed to be a caretaker.

–Roberta

I just feel like I have this responsibility to the community that I have to fulfill and that's just a part of me . . . I feel like I would be being irresponsible if I didn't do certain things I'm trying to do in the community.

–Jackie

There is a correlation between maybe our traditional role as I see it as two-spirited people and our relevance in healthcare . . . I mean we find our way into this nurturing society role and that we should really look at that as more of a traditional way to contribute to a society. Just like when we were home slaughtering buffalo and because we were the strong winkte [a tribally-specific term for two-spirit], we were cutting up the meat from the bone, from disconnecting the back leg of the buffalo and pulling it off and giving it to grandma to actually cut into smaller pieces you know? It's that concrete.

–Mary

A PRIMARY TWO-SPIRIT ROLE–
CARETAKING OF SICK AND ELDERLY PEOPLE

Through the interviews we learned that many of the respondents had cared for sick family, friends or elders. Although challenging, caregiving was commonly viewed as an accepted and even anticipated role for these two-spirit leaders. Further, caregiving was referenced as a larger Native community expectation of two-spirit people which they took pride in fulfilling.

> Caregiving is totally important, it's totally important to our two-spirit self, who we are . . . We had this wonderful guy in the community [that had been terribly abused as a child by his parents]. And then I watched him take care of those parents. And they had–I'm telling you, there's like 12 kids, but he is the one–and he's the two-spirited one, he's the only one. So he is taking care of those parents that were abusive to him, but yet because that is in our DNA as two-spirited people that we love our people. That he, despite all that happened to him, took care of that mother. I'm telling you, he was there. When she said frog, he jumped. Because he wanted to take care–and he took care of her up until the very end. And I went to the funeral when she passed and he wailed. And he hurt so bad. And now the father's still alive and he's taking care of him. It blows me away, it blows me away that tenderness, that love for each other.
>
> –Mary

> A dear friend of mine from my tribe is taking care of his grandmother. Nobody else will. So our people are constantly, constantly the ones that are relied upon. And I kept thinking, why is it just us–the two-spirits? Why is it not somebody else? And it was like Creator and the old ones told me it's because you all have such the love and the passion for people and the people see it. And we have such caringness, and that we love our people, that's why. It's just part of who we are. And I see it constantly. I look around the room, and I see everyone of our guys having one or the other part of caregiving in their family. Yeah, it's amazing. Totally.
>
> –Mary

I took care of my grandmothers, my great-grandmother . . . I mean they constantly wanted me to be with them. They constantly wanted me to take care of them. And I was constantly at my grandmother's house, and I was doing cooking, helping, being with her, making her laugh, my grandmother, my great-grandmother. It was so awesome to be able to know my great-grandmother. And I would sit on the porch with her and she would be churning butter the old fashioned way and I was the one and I think back, I was the only one that they called upon. And as they got older because my great-grandmother lived to be 98 and my grandmother lived to be 97, and up until the end they were calling for me . . . And it was just that, it was just that, oh it makes me teary. Because I miss them. Because we had such a bond together. And such a relationship. And I'd love to take care of them. I loved taking care of them [sniffs].

–Jackie

When I spoke earlier about sitting down with this elder woman and her just saying you know like, oh you're winkte [tribally specific word for two-spirit] and you can be a caregiver . . . and that's related to how I feel about our survival as a community you know . . . Maybe that's why I'm trying to return professionally to provide support to help people survive. So it's nurturing in that way.

–Al

I can't think of [any two-spirit person] that isn't, you know, that's not taking care of at least one, maybe two people.

–Marc

CAREGIVING FOR CHILDREN

It was even more common among respondents to have parented children and/or served as primary caregivers of children at some point. This was often viewed as an integral part of both their Native identities and their two-spirit identities.

And like we have a family model in our reservation which is extended, we don't have one mother, we have many mothers, many fathers, any uncle can be a father, any aunt can be a mother. It's very (enmeshed) and this makes my non-Native friends very uncomfortable when I go home and like we're sitting there and then an uncle will come in and just say hello and make himself at home like it's his house. So, those kinds of things traditionally, tribal living, kind of looking at that, but I really think we have to look at our role nationally in the larger picture because I think it will validate what we know traditionally.

–Mary

I think especially like older lesbians, we all have children, because we did what we thought was available . . . and those of us who didn't ended up taking care of other kids anyway . . .

–Roberta

A number of the respondents had been asked by family members to help raise children.

In terms of children, I was sterilized when I was seventeen. I wanted to have children, even though I knew I was a lesbian. By the government, I didn't know what was happening at the time, like a lot of young Native women. And um, I've helped raise my nephew and niece.

–Marie

My oldest sister was having problems, health problems and alcohol problems, and just a lot of marital problems and things, and she had two children and she was expecting a third one and she called me and she said, "You know, I can't take care of the kids. Would you be willing to take this new one that I'm going to have?" And I was kind of surprised and . . . I said "Yeah, but you have to remember, you have to understand, you know, my life too that I'm gay." And she said, "Oh, (JR)," she said, "I love you and I know you–we all love you." She says, "Don't worry about that. That's not a problem, just take care of him." . . . And I've had him since then . . . [At first I] stayed with my mom three weeks and she showed me how to take care of him and how to wrap him and change him and bathe him and all these things . . . I had a hard time sleeping at night 'cause you know there was crib death and all that stuff to think about, and I would nudge him and keep him awake. I cradle wrapped him all the time, for two years he was cradle wrapped. And uh, I'm surprised he's alive today! (laughs). He's 16, going to be 17.

–JR

And I actually a couple years ago, actually four or five years ago we [*my partner and I*] took my sister and I think she was like nine at the time, she came and I got custody of her for awhile. My mom was so supportive of it because she knew it was a good opportunity for her. So we had her come out here and she stayed with us for awhile and you know it's a huge responsibility for us but we were up for it and you know we moved into a bigger house so we could accommodate the extra body in the house. So she stayed with us for like eight months.

–Matt

My partner D. and I served as foster parents for a friend of ours. And so he lived with us for like three years. There isn't anything official there's no paperwork involved I mean, D. could walk in and say I'd like my son back, and we'd have to go okay, but to the extent she put up with it and, and, and he benefited from it, it worked.

–Camille

Notably, there was a sense in the interviews that raising children and helping to raise children was beneficial to the two-spirit community as a whole.

I know a lot of two-spirit people are parents or are taking on relatives' children, you know taking on cousins and raising children and that has an impact on them and that's changing the base of our (two-spirit) community for the good, I think.

–Terri

When we care for the children, we are a part of the heart of the community. Central to the whole Native community and that's helping us regain our traditional roles.

–Mary

MESSAGES RECEIVED ABOUT PARENTING/CAREGIVING

Respondents were asked about the messages they had received either explicitly or implicitly about being gay and being a parent–from family, from the Native community, from the LGBT community, or any other communities. Throughout the interviews, respondents highlighted the positive messages about being caregivers from family or Native community members.

I mean growing up I never heard anything but when we were going to take my sister on everybody was so supportive because they knew we were so responsible and together that they knew she would have a really good opportunity here. But everybody was so supportive. And then we took in my sister's baby and everybody again was pushing to have me get involved and get the baby 'cause they knew we could do it. And you know for me that was a good feeling' cause I was like, wow people aren't even thinking of anything, in a positive or negative way . . . It was just kind of–it's just the way it should be and they're accepting of it.

–JR

[People from my tribe] would be so supportive . . . I just went back last weekend to see my grandma' cause she's in the hospital. So when I came back she called and she was like, do you want to adopt a kid [interviewer laughs] because one of our cousins had her baby too young and blah blah blah blah and I'm like, no, you know I just can't think of that now, if I'm going to take the kid it's going to be for, you know, my niece. But you know, they're' already trying to push kids off on me, so I know that they would be very supportive [both laugh].

–Martin

I think [my family] would love it. I think they would adore that. They might not be comfortable with the situation [laughs] surrounding me having kids at first, but they would definitely come around. They better come around. [researcher laughs] . . . My dad might think it's a little crazy at first but he would be like whatever, that's great. I'm happy for you.

Interviewer: Okay, and how do you think you'd be received in the broader community?

Respondent: In the broader Native community that's what would matter, in the non-Native community it wouldn't matter but in the broader Native community, I would hope that they would be supportive and understanding and happy. I would hope that that's the response I would get. I'm sure they would. I think everybody, at least my friends in the Native community would be very happy for me.

Interviewer: So you wouldn't be impacted too much by what the non-Native community thought?

Respondent: No. Not one bit. Not one bit.

–Thomas

CAREGIVING SUPPORT FROM TWO-SPIRIT COMMUNITY

Some respondents discussed the challenges of caregiving and talked about the support they had received in this role. It was clear through the interviews that other two-spirit people played a primary role in easing the burdens related to caregiving.

I was a teen parent and without, without that I would not have been able to be an effective parent, um [clears throat] the resources and support that I was able to access were directly a result of my relationships with two-spirited Natives where I was living, you know, just I mean literally from feeding me and my kids for a year, standing in food lines for me, just you know everything you can think of, not being able to afford medicine and having them take care of that, um, just everything, and now it's interesting because my middle daughter is two-spirited and very uncomfortable with it, and so watching her struggle through that is something that I couldn't have done without having the two-spirit community around me in the first place to be able to support her through it. And then my older daughter, is a butterfly spirit and she has to be treated very tenderly and gingerly and she finds that with her two-spirited uncles and aunties. She just finds that nurturing, she can, she cannot access that in all of her communities, but she can when she's a (young kid) and wants to put her head in somebody's lap, that's the only place that she can go. That's it. And she's met other youth that have two-spirited parents or family members so that now she can be open and feel comfortable.

–Viv

My granddaughter has been with me now for the last six years and if it wasn't for the two-spirit community, I don't know if I would be alive.

–Terri

[My granddaughter] knows there's not just grandma, she's got aunties and men who care whatever happens to her. Everyone has her best intentions at heart . . . and so she's definitely a child that's being raised by the community.

–Roberta

DISCUSSION

The narratives in this study illustrate the critical role of two-spirits in providing caregiving across the lifespan to extended family members and kin within their communities. Caregiving is perceived as an important and integral role of two-spirit people, and it is clear that many two-spirit people already engage in caregiving or expect to provide care for others at some point during their lifetime. Importantly, the findings of this study demonstrate significant variability in the types of caregiving relationships that exist among two-spirit caregivers and their loved ones. Based on culturally proscribed roles, two-spirit people may be asked to care for the elderly, relatives, or children. In some communities, they may be asked to care for the community as a whole as they take on specific social or ceremonial responsibilities. In general, the people we interviewed spoke with pride about their caregiving responsibilities and a few noted how serving as a caregiver tied them to the Native community in an immediate and central way, particularly when they cared for children.

While much of the general caregiving literature focuses on caregiver burden, the people we interviewed often viewed caretaking as a challenging but central part of their two-spirit identity and role expectation. They literally would not be who they are as two-spirit people if separated from their caregiving roles. Yet, there are clearly also extra social, emotional, and financial burdens that accompany caregiving responsibilities and, as illustrated in the interviews, two-spirit people may take on caregiving roles at multiple levels (eg. individual and community) simultaneously.

Consistent with indigenous worldviews related to kinship systems and collective systems of care, several participants stressed the critical role of community support in assisting two-spirit caregivers and spoke to the need for more support; in particular, cultural systems of support (e.g., connection to extended family systems and other kinship structures of support). To insure that two-spirit individuals have access to appropriate support services, service providers must modify as necessary the accessibility and cultural relevance of community-based services assisting caregivers and their families (Fredriksen-Goldsen & Farwell, 2004). Negative experiences with health and social service systems and the absence of staff of similar cultural backgrounds (Cox & Monk, 1996; Gordon, 1995; Ortiz et al., 1999; Talamantes et al., 1995) need to be addressed to increase access to and utilization of services.

It is also important that service providers are cognizant of the tremendous tribal and cultural diversity reflected in the two-spirit population. When assessing needs, for example, providers must consider intra-cultural as well as intercultural differences related to help-seeking. Given the extent of caregiving and the range of caretaking activities discussed by respondents, concerted awareness programs are called for to educate organizations and agencies that support two-spirit people. Further, as so many of those interviewed were quite active in their Native communities, it is critical that organizations work with Native agencies in their efforts to reach out to two-spirit people and provide culturally meaningful services.

Many existing caregiver support programs and policies also reflect a cultural bias by only assisting caregivers who are providing support to elderly and immediate family members. Our findings suggest that two-spirit people may be more likely than others to parent or care for children or for non-relative community members. Indeed, caring for children or community needs may be an accepted and anticipated role for two-spirit people. Educating caregiver support programs on these practices is critical.

Finally, additional research is needed to more fully understand the needs and experiences of two-spirit as well as other caregivers in Native American communities. Often, two-spirit and other Native people are not included in caregiving research, limiting what we know about caregiving responsibilities in Native communities and related challenges. Indigenous worldviews regarding caregiving roles in relation to collective responsibility and systems of care need to be further developed in the caregiving literature to fully theorize and respond to issues related to caregiving burden and distress. Additionally, to build our knowledge base in this area, scholars and researchers must make concerted efforts to include two-spirit and Native people in their research and outreach efforts. Such a knowledge base will be critical in enabling family practitioners to more fully understand the range of experiences among ethnically diverse caregivers and to tailor services and policies to assist them and their families. Finally, expanding the caregiving knowledge base to include collective systems of care and indigenist worldviews will undoubtedly strengthen caregiving intervention development for diverse communities.

REFERENCES

Anguksuar [LaFortune, R]. (1997). A postcolonial perspective on Western [mis]conceptions of the cosmos and the restoration of indigenous taxonomies. In S. E. Jacobs, W. Thomas & S. Lang (Eds.), *Two-spirit people: Native American gender identity, sexuality, and spirituality* (pp. 217-222). Chicago: University of Illinois Press.

Bishop, R. (2005). Freeing ourselves from neocolonial domination in research: A Kaupapa Maori approach to creating knowledge. In N. Denzin and Y. S. Lincoln (Eds.), *The SAGE handbook of qualitative research, 3rd edition,* (pp. 109-138). Thousand Oaks, CA: Sage.

Brown, L. B. (1997). Women and men, not-men and not-women, lesbians and gays: American Indian gender style alternatives. *Journal of Gay and Lesbian Social Services, 6*(2), 5-20.

Cox, C., & Monk, A. (1996). Strain among caregivers: Comparing the experiences of African American and Hispanic caregivers of Alzheimer's relatives. *International Journal of Aging and Human Development, 43*(2), 93-106

Dilworth-Anderson, P., Williams, S.W., & Cooper, T. (1999). Family caregiving to elderly African Americans: Caregiver types and structures. *Journal of Gerontology: Social Sciences, 54B,* 237-241

Dilworth-Anderson, P., Williams, I. C., & Gibson, B. E. (2002). Issues of race, ethnicity, and culture in caregiving research: A 20-year review (1980-2000). *Gerontologist, 42*(2), 237-272

Farrer, C. A. (1997). Dealing with homophobia in everyday life. In S. E. Jacobs, W. T. Thomas, & S. Lang (Eds.), *Two-spirit people: Native American gender identity, sexuality, and spirituality* (pp.297-317).Chicago: University of Illinois Press.

Foley, K. L., Tung, H. J., Mutran, E. J. (2002). Self-gain and self-loss among African American and white caregivers. *Journals of Gerontology: Series B: Psychological Sciences and Social Sciences, 57*(1), 14-22.

Fredman, L., Daly, M. P. & Lazur, A. M. (1995). Burden among White and Black caregivers to elderly adults. *Journal of Gerontology, 50B*(2), 110-118.

Fredriksen-Goldsen, K. I., & Farwell, N. (2004). Dual responsibilities among Black, Hispanic, Asian and White caregivers: Implications for social work practice. *Journal of Gerontological Social Work, 4*(43), 25-44.

Gilligan, C., Spencer, R., Weinberg, M. K., & Bertsch, T. (2003). On the listening guide: A voice-centered relational method. In P. M. Camic, J. E. Rhodes, & L. Yardley (Eds.), *Qualitative research in psychology: Expanding perspectives in methodology and design* (pp. 157-172). Washington, DC: American Psychological Association.

Gitlin, L. N., Corcoran, M., Winter, L., Boyce, A., & Hauck, W. W. (2001). A randomized, controlled trial of a home environmental intervention: Effect on efficacy and upset in caregivers and on daily function of persons with dementia. *Gerontologist, 41*(1), 4-14.

Gordon, A. K. (1995). Deterrents to access and service for Blacks and Hispanics: The Medicare Hospice Benefit, healthcare utilization, and cultural barriers. *Hospice Journal, 10*(2), 65-83.

Henderson, J. N., & Traphagan, J. W. (2005). Cultural factors in dementia: Perspectives from the anthropology of aging. *Alzheimer's Disease and Associated Disorders, 19*(4), 272-274.

Hennessy, C. H., & John, R. (1995). The interpretation of burden among Pueblo Indian caregivers. *Journal of Aging Studies, 9*(3), 215–229.

Hennessy, C. H., & John, R. (1996). American Indian family caregivers' perceptions of burden and needed support. *Journal of Applied Gerontology, 15*(3), 275-294.

Hennessy, C. H., John, R., & Anderson, L. A. (1999). Diabetes education needs of family members caring for American Indian elders. *The Diabetes Educator, 25*, 747–754.

Hinrichsen, G. A. & Ramirez, M. (1992). Black and white dementia caregivers: A comparison of adaptation, adjustment and service utilization. *The Gerontologist, 32*(3), 375-381.

Jacobs, S.E., Thomas, W., & Lang, S. (1997). Introduction. In S. E. Jacobs, W. Thomas & S. Lang (Eds.), *Two-spirit people: Native American gender identity, sexuality, and spirituality* (pp. 1-18). Chicago: University of Illinois Press.

Jervis, L. L., & Manson, S. M. (2002). American Indians/Alaska Natives and dementia. *Alzheimer Disease and Associated Disorders, 16*(2), S89-95.

John, R., Hennessy, C. H., Dyeson, T., & Garrett, M. D. (2001). Toward the conceptualization and measurement of caregiver burden among Pueblo Indian family caregivers. *The Gerontologist, 41*(2), 410-419.

Lang, S. (1998). *Men as women, women as men: Changing gender in Native American cultures* (J. L. Vantine, Trans.). Austin: University of Texas Press.

Little Crow, Wright, J. A., & Brown, L. A. (1997). Gender selection in two American Indian tribes. *Journal of Gay and Lesbian Social Services, 6*(2), 21-28.

Martin, C.D. (2000). More than the work: Race and gender differences in caregiving burden. *Journal of Family Issues, 21*(8), 986-1005.

McCann, J. J., Hebert, L. E., Beckett, L. A., Morris, M. C., Scherr, P. A., & Evans, D. A. (2000). Comparison of informal caregiving by Black and White older adults in a community population. *Journal of the American Geriatrics Society, 48*(12), 1612-1679.

McMahon, E., & Rogers, K. L. (Eds.) (1994). *Interactive oral history interviewing.* Hillsdale, NJ: Lawrence Erlbaum.

Ortiz, A., Simmons, J., & Hinton, W. L. (1999). Locations of remorse and homelands of resilience: Notes on grief and sense of loss of place of Latino and Irish-American caregivers of demented elders. Culture, *Medicine and Psychiatry,* 23(4), 477-500.

Peck, M. K., Coward, R. T., Peck, C. W. (2000). Race, aging and care. *Research on Aging, 22*(2), 117-143.

Strong, C. (1984). Stress and caring for elderly relatives: Interpretations and coping strategies in an American Indian and White sample. *The Gerontologist, 24,* 251-256.

Talamantes, M., Lawler, W. R., & Espino, D. V. (1995). Hispanic American elders: Caregiving norms surrounding dying and the use of hospice services. *Hospice Journal, 10*(2), 35-49.

Thomas, W., & Jacobs, S. E. (1999). ". . . And we are still here": From *berdache* to two-spirit people. *American Indian Culture and Research Journal, 23*(2), 91-107.

Thornton, M. C. (1998). Indigenous resources and strategies of resistance: Informal caregiving and racial socialization in Black communities. In H. I. McCubbin (Ed), *Resiliency in African American families.* Resiliency in Families Series, Vol. 3. (49-66). Thousand Oaks, Ca: Sage Publications.

Tinker, G. E.(1993). *Missionary conquest: The gospel and Native American cultural genocide.* Minneapolis:Fortress Press.

Tuhiwai Smith, L. (2005). On tricky ground: Researching the Native in the age of uncertainty. In N. Denzin & Y. S. Lincoln (Eds.), *The SAGE handbook of qualitative research, 3rd edition,* (pp. 85-107). Thousand Oaks, CA: Sage.

Walters, K., Evans-Campbell, T., Simoni, J., Ronquillo, T., & Bhuyan, R. (2006). "My Spirit in My Heart": Identity experiences and challenges among American Indian Two-Spirit Women. *Journal of Lesbian Studies, 10*(1/2), 125-149.

Yates, M. E., Tennstedt, S., & Chang, B. H. (1999). Contributors to and mediators of psychological well-being for informal caregivers. *The Journals of Gerontology: Series B: Psychological Sciences and Social Sciences, 54B*(1), 12-23.

Young, R. F., & Kahana, E. (1995). The context of caregiving and well-being outcomes among African and Caucasian Americans. *The Gerontologist,* 35(2), 225-232.

doi:10.1300/J041v18n03_05

Transgender Health:
Implications for Aging and Caregiving

Mark E. Williams
Pat A. Freeman

SUMMARY. Transgender people face many typical experiences associated with growing old compounded by unique stresses and challenges related to being transgender. Public and corporate policies and a history of discrimination tend to isolate transgender elders, potentially impairing their health, quality of life, and longevity. Health care providers and transgender people alike need accurate and representative information about the experiences and needs of these elders. Research on the lives and concerns of transgender elders is necessary to better understand their aging and caregiving experiences and to illuminate effective and respectful interventions to support them across the life course. doi:10.1300/ J041v18n03_06 *[Article copies available for a fee from The Haworth Document Delivery Service: 1-800-HAWORTH. E-mail address: <docdelivery@ haworthpress.com> Website: <http://www.HaworthPress.com> © 2007 by The Haworth Press, Inc. All rights reserved.]*

KEYWORDS. Transgender, trans, gender identity, FTM, MTF, health, aging, caregiving

Mark E. Williams is affiliated with the School of Social Work, University of Washington, Seattle, WA.

Pat A. Freeman is Historian, Northwest LGBT History Project, Seattle, WA.

[Haworth co-indexing entry note]: "Transgender Health: Implications for Aging and Caregiving." Williams, Mark E., and Pat A. Freeman. Co-published simultaneously in *Journal of Gay & Lesbian Social Services* (The Haworth Press, Inc.) Vol. 18, No. 3/4, 2007, pp. 93-108; and: *Caregiving with Pride* (ed: Karen I. Fredriksen-Goldsen) The Haworth Press, Inc., 2007, pp. 93-108. Single or multiple copies of this article are available for a fee from The Haworth Document Delivery Service [1-800-HAWORTH, 9:00 a.m. - 5:00 p.m. (EST). E-mail address: docdelivery@haworthpress.com].

INTRODUCTION

Indications are that the transgender aging population will continue to grow. Yet, transgender health, aging and caregiving are understudied fields of inquiry with only preliminary research to date. Current research on transgender health still relies primarily on extrapolation from previous studies of gay men, lesbians and bisexual persons (GLBs) that do not necessarily reflect issues of concern to transgender elders. Information about transgender caregiving, particularly as it relates to health and aging issues, is essentially non-existent.

Many articles and studies have summarized conclusions about the "LGBT community" (lesbian, gay, bisexual and transgender), while citing research and discussing conclusions that in fact only directly address lesbians and gay men, and to a lesser extent, bisexual individuals. While some transgender issues overlap with research about GLB concerns, such as the need for health care, research continues to neglect issues specific to the lives of some transgender persons, such as transitioning. In this paper we will begin by reviewing transgender history; within that context, we will then review existing literature about transgender health, discussing its potential implications for aging and caregiving.

HISTORICAL CONTEXT

Lesbian and gay history now has a fairly extensive research base. The same, however, cannot be said for transgender history, although since the late 1800s transgender history does, to a degree, parallel gay and lesbian history. Sexual activities between adults, especially gay and lesbian activities, were generally of little interest to the heterosexual population until the 1890s, when sexologists such as Kraft-Ebbing and Havelock Ellis began examining homosexuality and transgenderism from a medical model. What might be called 'robust' platonic relationships between men and romantic friendships and Boston marriages between women, once looked upon with favor by society, were now viewed as evidence of undesirable, immoral, and abnormal behavior. Public sentiment held that men and women who indulged in such debauchery should be medically cured or incarcerated. There were social and legal consequences for such behavior, especially for the easily labeled effeminate male and masculine female. After homosexual acts began to be pathologized via the medical model, states rapidly added sodomy to their list of punishable sex acts, which already included activities such as adultery, prostitution and "wanton" behavior (Atkins, 2003).

To avoid legal and social penalties, gay men, lesbians and bisexual persons sought protection by becoming invisible to heterosexual society and developing underground and closeted lives. Many who today would probably be referred to as transgender quietly "passed" and went about their lives. Some transgender people successfully lived and worked as genders other than those associated with their biological sex. For gay men, lesbians, bisexual and transgender persons (GLBTs), passing in socially acceptable roles became essential to survival, safety and quality of life (Sullivan, 1990). With the increasing enforcement of sodomy laws, especially from the 1930s on, GLBT invisibility became standard practice in mainstream society.

Evelyn Hooker was one of the first researchers to empirically challenge the accepted belief of the psychiatric and medical professions that gay men were neurotic, often bordering on psychotic, afflicted with numerous nervous symptoms, immature, and incapable of functioning satisfactorily in society. In Hooker's (1957) study of 30 gay men and 30 heterosexual men, she determined that gay men were as well adjusted as heterosexual men, and in fact in some respects were better adjusted. Still, it was not until 1973 that homosexuality was removed from the Diagnostic and Statistical Manual of Mental Disorders (Drescher, 2006). Around the same time, the transgender community was saddled with the diagnostic term "gender dysphoria syndrome," later called gender identity disorder. Gender identity disorder remains a psychiatric diagnosis in the Diagnostic and Statistical Manual today (American Psychiatric Association, 2000; Meyerowitz, 2002).

Christine Jorgensen's sex reassignment surgery (performed in Denmark in 1953) sparked the U. S. public's first mass media experience involving trangenderism. Largely ignorant of gender identity issues, most of the heterosexual public assumed that sex reassignment surgery was related to homosexuality and was merely a last resort for men who love men (Meyerowitz, 2002; Cook-Daniels, 2006). The U.S. medical community, itself divided over the issues surrounding sex reassignment surgery, did little to enlighten the public. The debate concerning whether the U.S. medical community should endorse such surgeries served largely to further pathologize and marginalize transgender people. For example, the conservative faction of the American Medical Association endorsed a law against sex reassignment surgery, based on old English common law that outlawed the maiming of any man who might become a soldier (Meyerowitz, 2002). Many physicians cited personal beliefs or fear of lawsuits as the basis for their refusal to perform any kind of surgery that could be construed as sex reassignment. The result was that some desperate men took matters, literally, into their own hands and performed their own castrations (Brevard, 2001).

Such drastic measures could be avoided if one had an income that would accommodate traveling to Europe for sex reassignment surgery. In general, due to the income disparity between men and women, as well as other factors, more men than women had sex reassignment surgery. However in practice, most men, like most women, did not have the financial means for such surgeries, and many simply did not want them. Instead, many intentionally expressed their gender identity and transgenderism as part of the gay community (Paulson, 1996). Others continued to choose the invisibility of the closet, living on the fringe of GLB or transgender communities or simply passing within heterosexual society.

As the transgender population grew in the late 1970s and early 1980s, health care providers and social service agencies became aware that transgender issues and concerns presented a growing challenge. Little information was available regarding transgender health and unique needs for specialized care. As a result, health care providers and social service agencies sought answers within the more widely examined GLB research. Many early conclusions about transgender health and health care were based on the assumption that the transgender community was simply a subset of the larger GLBT community with similar health issues. Evidence regarding the experiences and needs of gay men, lesbians and bisexual persons was extrapolated on the assumption that transgender health issues would be similar. These early efforts, however well intentioned, failed to reflect actual transgender health needs and concerns.

Within the past few years, transgender issues have increasingly become part of the public discourse and more information on gender identity is available to the public. For example, transgender concerns are now more openly addressed in the popular media such as television, movies (e.g., the 2006 box office hit "Transamerica") and books. New media technologies have provided unprecedented access to information and insights about transgender persons, old and young, and the rapidly evolving ways in which gender is expressed. An explosion of resources on transgender issues over the Internet has allowed those seeking more information and support to be connected with one another (Cook-Daniels, 2006).

Concurrent with this growing familiarity with transgender issues, a number of jurisdictions have recently passed anti-discrimination measures which include gender identity and expression. For example, Cincinnati (Ohio), Lansdowne and Swarthmore (Pennsylvania), Bloomington (Indiana), King County (Washington State), and Washington state itself all approved such bills in 2006 (Transgender Law & Policy Institute, 2006). While an increasing number of jurisdictions are enacting such legislation (National Center on Transgender Equality, 2006), the majority of Americans remain unprotected from discrimination based on gender identity.

Today, the transgender population is growing both in numbers and visibility, and includes an age range broader than in decades past. Youth are expressing non-conforming gender identities at a younger age, and transgender adults are living openly into old age. Yet many of the stereotypes and social patterns of past generations continue to be cited as the bases for understanding today's transgender population. Particularly when addressing the experiences of transgender older adults, outdated stereotypes and preconceptions often lead to erroneous conclusions that fail to identify issues and concerns pertinent to the current transgender population.

TRANSGENDER HEALTH

While a small body of literature examining transgender health experiences and aging has recently begun to be established, it remains limited in scope and quantity. Feldman and Bockting (2003) report that as many as 30% to 40% of transgender persons in the United States do not have a regular physician and often rely on emergency room and urgent care physicians for immediate health care needs. Thus, it seems that many transgender persons simply live with untreated or under-treated chronic conditions such as hypertension or diabetes. Furthermore, fear of revealing their transgender status may prevent adequate health screenings, such as for breast or prostate cancers. Treatable health conditions may increase in severity unnecessarily, due to the reluctance of transgender people, young and old, to either put themselves in further abusive situations or be forced to confront prejudice in the health care system (Cahill, South, & Spade, 2000). This may be particularly true for transgender elders who were part of a generation that was raised to passively accept the authority of medical professionals.

In general, transgender people face a number of barriers to accessing adequate health care. Violence, harassment, and discrimination are common experiences among transgender people, and they set the stage for particular challenges to health (Xavier et al., 2004; Lombardi, 2001). "Social and economic marginalization resulting from the pathologization of transgenderism means that access to health care and health insurance is even less prevalent among transgender individuals" than among gay, lesbian and bisexual individuals (Cahill et al., 2000, p. 13). Transgender people of color may be the most at risk for inadequate health care and health insurance coverage due to compounding sources of stigmatization and discrimination related to racism, transphobia, and poverty (Xavier et al., 2004; Cahill et al., 2000).

Underinsurance and lack of health insurance appear common, as joblessness and poverty are prevalent in transgender populations, particularly among people of color and youth (Xavier et al., 2004; Clement-Nolle, Marx, Guzman & Katz, 2001). Those who possess health insurance often find barriers to accessing their health benefits. Hong (2003) details how insurance companies rely on non-medical and non-fiscal criteria to exclude transition-related medical treatment from being covered under public or private insurance benefits. Most health insurance policies exclude coverage for transgender-specific health procedures, such as hormone therapy and sex reassignment surgery.

As a result, some transgender people may use unregulated or "off-label" medications, often obtained and used without medical supervision, and at times administered with shared needles, greatly increasing risk of HIV and hepatitis infections (Xavier et al., 2004; Feldman & Bockting, 2003; Lombardi, 2001; Clement-Nolle et al., 2001). Particularly among transgender women of color, there is widespread use of injection silicone as a cheap alternative to hormone therapy. Continued use of injection silicone can lead to illness, disfigurement and possibly death (Xavier et al., 2004).

Hormone therapy has the potential for many drug interactions, making unsupervised self-treatment even more dangerous, particularly for people being treated for illness or injuries by doctors who are unaware of the hormone therapy. Hormone therapy makes medically unsupervised self-treatment a high risk factor for a host of complications and further challenges to transgender health; it is associated with a higher risk for diabetes, cardiovascular disease, thromboembolic events, and liver abnormalities (Feldman & Bockting, 2003).

Testosterone therapy for female-to-male transgender men has, in some cases, been associated with an increased risk of heart disease, loss of bone density, endometrial hyperplasia and subsequent endometrial carcinoma (Futterwiet, 1998), and higher red blood cell count, which can be life threatening (Witten, Eyler & Wiegel, 2004). Male-to-female transgender women taking estrogen may face increased risk of type II diabetes, increased cholesterol, blood clots, loss of bone density, neo-vaginal cancer, and prostate cancer (Feldman & Bockting, 2003). Many transgender elders may be at greater risk than those who are younger because of the longer duration of hormone use, which may well exacerbate the effects of aging such as cardiac or pulmonary problems. More research is also needed to examine the potential risks associated with hormone use among transgender youth, especially prepubescent children.

Existing public policies have sanctioned and institutionalized the exclusion of transgender people from access to adequate health coverage and care. Prior to its passage, the Americans with Disabilities Act was explicitly amended, "denying protection for conditions related to gender dysphoria" (Hong, 2003, p. 1). As a result, insurance companies have routinely denied transgender consumers coverage for many transgender-specific health procedures such as hormone therapy and sex reassignment surgery.

The effects of the Americans with Disabilities Act exclusion clause percolate through the healthcare system as a whole. "Most disturbing, many insurers liberally apply the SRS (sex reassignment surgery) exclusion clause to deny transsexuals coverage for non-transition related, medically necessary conditions such as back pain, intestinal cysts, and even cancer, under the rationale that any medical care a transsexual needs is an excludable transsexual-related condition" (Hong, 2003, p. 2). Insurance companies have denied transgender consumers coverage for routine medical treatments, including office visits, blood tests, physical exams, sinus medication, and emergency visits, based on the exclusion of sex reassignment surgery.

Discrimination against transgender people in the health care system is not limited to insurers. Some physicians refuse to treat transgender patients. Other physicians who treat transgender patients persist in referring to them by their non-requested pronoun. Transgender health care consumers describe doctors, nurses, and emergency medical technicians responding with discomfort or disgust to their gender identity, including cracking jokes, insulting clients, and providing inadequate care (Drabble, Keatley, & Marcelle, 2003).

Some hospitals prevent transgender patients' own physicians from administering procedures to their patients. Doctors have been reported for refusing to administer gynecological care for female-to-male transgender people, including treatment of cervical cancer or abnormal vaginal discharges (Hong, 2003). Many transgender individuals who have repeatedly been barred from receiving medical care and treated disrespectfully by health care professionals subsequently delay seeking necessary care, thus putting themselves at unnecessary risk.

Effective communication is further complicated by cross-cultural issues of all types, including differences between non-transgender and transgender communities, as well as racial, ethnic and cultural differences between health care providers and transgender health care consumers. When willing medical care has been found, it often has required that transgender health care consumers educate their providers in culturally appropriate care. In some cases transgender patients find themselves educating their providers about specific needs and concerns related to transgender health care provision (Drabble et al., 2003).

It should be noted, however, that some gains have been made in transgender health policy, and that not all transgender people find access to adequate health care insurmountable. In 1999, the American Public Health Association passed its first resolution on transgender health issues in order to improve the treatment experienced by transgender persons seeking healthcare (Lombardi, 2001). Many individuals report that their doctors and employers have successfully advocated against insurers' denial of health coverage, and a minority of health insurance providers does cover all medical care needs of transgender people, including transition-related treatments (Hong, 2003). Surveys at one university sexual health clinic found consistently high rates of transgender patient satisfaction, comparable to the satisfaction rates of other health clinic patients (Bockting, Robinson, Benner, & Scheltema, 2004).

In addition to unique physical health needs, transgender people also appear to be at higher risk for some mental health concerns. One study (Clement-Nolle et al., 2001) of 392 transgender individuals found that about one-third of them had attempted suicide, which is a rate significantly higher than the general population and also higher than estimated rates for lesbians and gay men. Almost two-thirds of the male-to-female and 55% of the female-to-male participants were clinically depressed at the time of the study. Drabble et al. (2003) report transgender persons are at higher risk for compromised mental health as a result of discrimination, shame, isolation and sexual identity conflict.

Accessing mental health care is also a unique challenge for many transgender people. Mental health counselor bias has been detrimental to transgender clients. For example, some counselors have been shown to exert bias in counseling that includes pressuring clients into either/or decisions regarding gender, trying to talk clients out of gender reassignment, pushing clients prematurely to come out and identify as their internal gender, or pathologizing transgender identity as simply internalized homophobia (Drabble et al., 2003; Carroll & Gilroy, 2002; Craft, 2001).

Receiving effective mental health care is also complicated for many transgender individuals due to the dual role that many mental health professionals have in their work with transgender clients. Mental health professionals have held roles as gatekeepers to gender-transition treatments including hormone therapy and sex reassignment surgeries. This has undermined the potential for forming a trusting counseling relationship for many transgender people and at times engendered outright hostility toward mental health professionals as a whole (Bockting et al., 2004; Drabble et al., 2003; Carroll & Gilroy, 2002).

The current literature on transgender physical and mental health does not address cultural distinctions within the transgender population. For example, little is known about differences by race or ethnicity, class or socio-economic status, or immigrant or rural transgender experiences or health concerns. Research on transgender health has relied on non-random studies, and sexual health clinics have typically been used to recruit study participants. In addition, approaches to examining transgender health to date are problem-focused and fail to illuminate potentially unique sources of strength, coping and resilience in the transgender community that may buffer some of the disadvantages faced due to systemic oppression. Furthermore, we do not know whether commonly used interventions are actually effective for the transgender community. Clinicians often provide health and mental health care assuming that the treatments that have been validated for other populations will be efficacious for transgender persons; to date, however, that assumption is most often empirically unfounded.

Gender bias also appears to skew current transgender health research. To date male-to-female (MTF) transgender women are overrepresented in the current literature, and the experiences and needs of female-to-male (FTM) transgender men remain relatively unknown. In recent years the number of female-to-male (FTM) transgender men is increasing, but is still smaller than the population of male-to-female (MTF)/ transgender persons, whose higher numbers likely exert an influence on the findings of transgender health studies (Rosario, 2006).

Until national survey data include gender identity demographics, and social norms permit transgender individuals in all settings to self-identify safely and with dignity, conclusions about the unique challenges and resources for transgender health will remain preliminary. Even with broader inclusion of survey data, researchers and health providers must educate themselves regarding changes taking place in the transgender community. Yet to date, most new information regarding transgender health is not reaching health practitioners or researchers, and a vigorous re-education program needs to be undertaken.

TRANSGENDER AGING

Just as data about the transgender population as a whole is inconclusive, information about transgender elders is even more lacking. In general, elders in the United States face considerable challenges to healthy living as they grow old. For example, lack of long-term care insurance is impoverishing many elders; the cost of living and access to long-term care is putting health and security out of reach (Cahill et al., 2000). Elder research has shown a significant association between living alone and increased risk of lower income, poorer nutrition, decreased mental health, and risk for institutionalization (McMahon, 2003). Morrow (2004) points out that increased isolation is associated with low self-esteem, limited social skill development, substance abuse, and depression; all are exacerbated by limited financial resources.

An articulation of such needs, and how they will evolve as the transgender population ages, is not yet available. Convenience sampling from such sources as street clinics has skewed what little data is available, failing to adequately or accurately describe the diversity of transgender experiences and concerns. As a result, like early GLB research, transgender health studies have tended to focus on health issues and needs of younger transgender persons. Transgender elders remain largely invisible and their health and aging needs are not adequately examined in current literature.

Risk factors associated with growing old may be particularly pronounced for transgender elders. "Anecdotal evidence indicates that poverty and wage discrimination are widespread experiences of transgender people" in general, and transgender elders in particular (Cahill et al., 2000, p. 9). Gender disparities disproportionately impact the financial resources of some transgender elders more than others. "Incomes well below the U.S. national average are common among FTMs. Because many FTMs begin their transition only after years of lesbian identification–this is most likely a result of discrimination they experienced as women and lesbians" (Witten et al., 2004). Thus, there may be increasing reliance on public and social services for care and assistance as transgender persons age, making them more dependent on transphobic institutions, peers and family members.

Cahill et al. (2000) document discrimination, abuse and neglect of LGBT elders in nursing homes. Similarly, Johnson and Jackson (2005) confirm that a sample of gay, lesbian, bisexual and transgender elders experience considerable fear of discrimination in retirement and elder care facilities. Experiences of discrimination and the fear of discrimination collude to negatively impact the health and available resources for transgender elders. As they grow old and rely more heavily on public programs and health and social services for assistance, they may have less independence from heterosexist institutions. While LGBT senior housing projects are being built in several U.S. metropolitan areas, the extremely limited number of units that these projects represent will mostly be accessible to the very wealthy. Poor and middle class transgender elders will likely not find housing available in retirement facilities explicitly designed for GLBT communities for many years to come, potentially exacerbating the risk factors associated with elder isolation (Cahill & South, 2002).

Fear of experiencing discrimination can exacerbate social isolation, placing people at higher risk for decreases in quality and length of life (Cahill et al., 2000). Advocacy groups have recently begun programs to address discrimination, harassment and abuse of LGBT elders. For example, the Policy Institute of the National Gay and Lesbian Task Force launched its first aging initiative in 1999, devoting resources and scholarship to advocate for the needs of GLBT elders. The National Center for Lesbian Rights also recently began an aging initiative to provide free legal advice to GLBT elders. The Lambda Legal Defense and Education Fund similarly initiated an effort to identify and combat discrimination against LGBT elders.

The multiple challenges that transgender individuals face as they grow old come not only from mainstream heterosexual society. Transgender elders also may face ageism, racism, ableism, and other types of oppression that compound isolation and stressors for many transgender individuals. Cahill et al. (2000) describe transgender communal norms, similar to GLB norms, which emphasize youth and youthful beauty perhaps even more than heterosexual culture does. Ageism has, until recently, excluded elder issues from LGBT political agendas and the LGBT media, and resulted in few intergenerational LGBT organizations. Groups such as Old Lesbians Organizing for Change, Senior Action in a Gay Environment, and Pride Senior Network have organized to address ageism within LGBT communities and confront its impact.

Generational differences and dialogue within the transgender community pose another important area of inquiry that requires collaborative partnerships and foundational research to examine transgender issues across the lifespan.

Transgender individuals may possess unique resilience in the face of multiple challenges in their elder years. Cahill and South (2002) suggest that some transgender elders' experiences of discrimination during their middle adult years prepare them to better respond to the stresses of getting old. Having struggled in the face of transphobia prior to older adulthood, transgender elders may have unique tools that strengthen and equip them to endure multiple challenges associated with aging. Identifying the nature of this potential resilience and these unique coping tools will require further research.

Scholarly research regarding aging and the transgender community remains very limited. Much of what has been written about transgender aging issues is again based on extrapolation from research examining heterosexual and LGB elders. Little hard data on transgender elders exists, and the conclusions are tentative at best. Yet, increasingly transgender issues are becoming subjects of inquiry and scholarship. As researchers commit to exploring the experiences of transgender elders, we will deepen our understanding of the challenges and resources transgender individuals face as they age, and how these challenges and resources compare with those faced by other diverse populations.

TRANSGENDER CAREGIVING

The limited material that has been written regarding transgender caregiving is generally based on anecdotal evidence and conjecture. Although some conclusions appear reasonable, further research is needed to examine the experiences of both transgender caregivers and care recipients, and to understand the impact of gender identity on caregiving relationships and experiences.

Cahill et al. (2000) propose some assumptions about transgender caregiving, citing that most seniors turn to their families of origin for support and assistance. Specifically spouses, daughters and daughters-in-law provide most of the caregiving in the United States. If the trends evident among lesbian and gay elders are similar (or more pronounced) for transgender elders, then social isolation from family and lack of social support may place transgender elders at risk when they need care. If familial support is absent and access to child or spousal caregivers is not readily available to some transgender persons, they may frequently need to turn to public and fee-for-service assistance when they face debilitating effects of serious illness or functional impairment.

Fear of discrimination may serve as a barrier to transgender elders accessing necessary health care and assistance. "Of particular concern is what happens when a transgender person with a non-congruent body (meaning that an uninformed observer would think that the genitals or other physical features of a person do not 'match' the gender and/or legal identity) has to be intimately assisted by healthcare providers and caregivers, such as with bathing" (Cahill et al., 2000, p. 17). The need for assistance may place many transgender persons in the hands of family members and institutions that may be hostile to their gender identities. Due to lack of existing research, we do not know if such caregiving arrangements will result in increased interpersonal conflict, abuse, neglect, or intrapsychic stress from retreating to the closet.

Also unknown is whether transgender persons who require caregiving have success in finding more healthy, alternative sources of assistance when needed. Affirming and respectful caregiving under the best of circumstances presents stress and difficulties to both caregivers and care recipients. Transgender caregivers and caregivers for transgender persons may not fit into traditional definitions of "family," and they may face obstacles to obtaining information from or being acknowledged by hospital and nursing home staff. Mail and Safford (2003) suggest that caregivers of HIV positive transgender people may find spirituality as a source of growth, value, and direction that promotes their well-being as they cope with the stress of providing care. Other resources and sources of strength for transgender people involved in caregiving relationships have yet to be fully investigated.

Further research is needed in all aspects of transgender caregiving. In particular, research is needed to understand what caregiving arrangements transgender elders are currently creating for themselves, and whether fear and anticipation of discrimination is causing them to delay accessing necessary assistance. For example, are transgender elders choosing to become closeted in order to secure needed assistance? For all members of the transgender community, an education program is needed that includes components of elder law such as wills, power of attorney, health directives, estate planning, anti-discrimination laws, and referrals for legal assistance.

CONCLUSION

Transgender people not only face common health issues typical to the general population, but also unique health challenges arising from discrimination, stigmatization, isolation and inattention. In particular, they require knowledgeable and respectful health care provided by professionals who are responsive to general health concerns and also understand the unique health challenges that transgender people face. Despite evidence that transgender persons face unique health issues, they are almost entirely absent from studies regarding physical and mental health treatments (Meyer, 2001; Carroll, Gilroy, & Ryan, 2002).

Education regarding transgender health and aging is called for at all levels of society. From health care providers and caregivers to transgender people themselves, accurate, representative information about the experiences and needs of diverse transgender elders is needed. Transgender elders face the typical stresses of growing old compounded by unique stresses and challenges related to being transgender. Federal laws, public and private policies, and violent and dehumanizing discrimination collude to isolate transgender elders and potentially impair their health, quality of life, and longevity. Lack of health insurance coverage and inadequate health care exacerbate the unique health challenges that transgender persons encounter.

Today more individuals are openly identifying themselves as transgender or gender non-conforming. Many are prevailing over the challenges placed before them, as they are growing in visibility and influence in society. While transphobic oppression is an obstacle, transgender people are carving out a public identity and claiming their rights as full members of society. The preliminary research on transgender lives and aging suggests that despite the obstacles present, transgender people are moving forward to shape their lives with dignity and self-determination.

It is time to establish an empirical base to paint a more detailed and vivid picture of the needs and resilience of transgender elders. Because of the rapid increase in the size of the transgender community, particularly the aging population, a renewed call for in-depth research on current health and quality of life issues is timely. Practitioners, scholars and funding sources alike must step up to insure effective services and rigorous research that will be positioned to have a powerful impact in shaping policies and improving the lives of transgender elders.

REFERENCES

American Psychiatric Association (2000). *Diagnostic and Statistical Manual of Mental Disorders*, (4th ed.), Text Revision. Washington, DC: Author.

Atkins, G. L. (2003). *Gay Seattle: Stories of exile and belonging*. Seattle: University of Washington Press.

Bockting, W. O., Robinson, B. E., Benner, A., & Scheltema, K. (2004). Patient satisfaction with transgender health services. *Journal of Sex and Marital Therapy. 30*(4), 277-294.

Brevard, A. (2001). *The woman I was not born to be*. Philadelphia: Temple University Press.

Cahill, S., South, K., & Spade, J. (2000). *Outing age: Public policy issues affecting gay, lesbian, bisexual and transgender elders*. Washington, DC: The Policy Institute of the National Gay and Lesbian Task Force Foundation. Retrieved May 31, 2006 from http://www.thetaskforce.org/downloads/outingage.pdf.

Cahill, S., & South, K. (2002). Policy issues affecting lesbian, gay, bisexual, and transgender people in retirement. *Generations, 26*(2), 49-54.

Carroll, L. & Gilroy, P .J. (2002). Transgender issues in counselor preparation. *Counselor Education and Supervision, 41*(3), 233-242.

Carroll, L., Gilroy, P. J., & Ryan, J. (2002). Counseling transgendered, transsexual, and gender-variant clients. *Journal of Counseling and Development, 80*(2), 131-139.

Clement-Nolle, K., Marx, R., Guzman, R., & Katz, M. (2001). HIV prevalence, risk behaviors, health care use, and mental health status of transgender persons: Implications for public health intervention. *American Journal of Public Health, 91*(6), 915-921.

Cook-Daniels, L. (2006). Trans aging. In D. Kimmel, T. Rose, & S. David (Eds.), *Lesbian, gay, bisexual, and transgender aging: Research and clinical perspectives*. New York: Columbia University Press.

Craft, E. M. (2001). Addressing lesbian, gay, bisexual, and transgender issues from the inside: One federal agency's approach. *American Journal of Public Health, 91*(6), 889-891.

Drabble, L., Keatley, J., & Marcelle, G. (2003). Progress and opportunities in lesbian, gay, bisexual, and transgender health communications. *Clinical Research and Regulatory Affairs, 20*(2), 205-227.

Drescher, J. (2006). An interview with Robert L. Spitzer, MD. In J. Drescher & K. J. Zucker (Eds.), *Ex-Gay research: Analyzing the Spitzer study and its relation to science, religion, politics, and culture*. (pp. 323-339). Binghamton, NY: Harrington Park Press/Haworth Press.

Feldman, J., & Bockting, W. (2003). Transgender health. *Minnesota Medicine, 86*(7), 25-32.

Futterwiet, W. (1998). Endocrine therapy of transsexualism and potential complications of long-term treatment. *Archives of Sexual Behavior, 27*, 209-226.

Hong, K. E. (2003). Categorical exclusions: Exploring legal responses to health care discrimination against transsexuals. *Columbia Journal of Gender and Law, 14*(1).

Hooker, E. (1957). The adjustment of the male overt homosexual. *Journal of Projective Techniques, 21*, 18-31.

Johnson, M. J., & Jackson, N. C. (2005). Gay and lesbian perceptions of discrimination in retirement care facilities. *Journal of Homosexuality, 42*(2), 83-102.

Lombardi, E. (2001). Enhancing transgender health care. *American Journal of Public Health, 91*(6), 869-872.

Mail, P. D., & Safford, L. (2003). LGBT disease prevention and health promotion: Wellness for gay, lesbian, bisexual, and transgender individuals and communities. *Clinical Research and Regulatory Affairs, 20*(2), 183-204.

McMahon, E. (2003). The older homosexual: Current concepts of lesbian, gay, bisexual, and transgender older Americans. *Clinics in Geriatric Medicine, 19*, 587-593.

Meyer, I. H. (2001). Why lesbian, gay, bisexual and transgender public health? *American Journal of Public Health, 91*(6), 856-859.

Meyerowitz, J. (2002). *How sex changed: A history of transsexuality in the United States.* Cambridge: Harvard University Press.

Morrow, D. (2004). Social work practice with gay, lesbian, bisexual, and transgender adolescents. *Families in Society, 85*(1), 91-99.

National Center for Transgender Equality. (2006). Retrieved June 13, 2006, from http://www.ncte.org

Paulson, D. (with Simpson, R.). (1996). *An evening at the Garden of Allah: A gay cabaret in Seattle.* New York: Columbia University Press.

Rosario, V. (2006). Can science explain gender nonconformity. *The Gay & Lesbian Review, 13*(3), pp 39-42.

Sullivan, L. (1990). *From female to male: The life of Jack Bee Garland.* Boston: Alyson Publications, Inc.

Transgender Law & Policy Institute. (2006). *Scope of explicitly transgender-inclusive anti-discrimination laws.* Retrieved June 22, 2006, from http://www.transgenderlaw.org

Witten, T. M., Eyler, A. E. & Wiegel, C. (2004). *Trans issues in aging: Information for health care providers.* Retrieved May 31, 2006, from http://www.temenos.net/articles/05-02-04.shtml.

Xavier, J., Hitchcock, D., Hollinshead, S., Keisling, M., Lewis, Y., Lombardi, E., et al. (2004). *An overview of U.S. trans health priorities: A report by the Eliminating Disparities Working Group.* National Coalition for LGBT Health: Washington, DC.

doi:10.1300/J041v18n03_06

Exploring Interventions for LGBT Caregivers: Issues and Examples

David W. Coon

SUMMARY. LGBT caregiving for midlife and older adults facing chronic illness or disability as well as the development and evaluation of interventions targeting LGBT caregivers remains fundamentally unexplored. Caregivers regardless of their sexual orientation or gender identity often juggle multiple roles and responsibilities leading to increased stress and distress. However, largely due to discrimination and discriminatory policies, many LGBT caregivers face barriers at multiple levels of service provision that can exacerbate stress and negatively impact caregiver and care recipient quality of life. This article highlights many of these obstacles and provides examples of intervention strategies designed to assist LGBT caregivers ranging from interventions aimed at the individual and interpersonal levels of service provision to changes needed at the social policy level. As an example of an individual or interpersonal level of intervention designed to assist LGBT caregivers, the SURE 2 framework is presented and more thoroughly discussed. Given the diversity of the LGBT community, the article ends with ways to extend or adapt SURE 2 as well as suggesting that the time has come to develop and test a variety of interventions for LGBT caregivers. doi:10.1300/J041v18n03_07 *[Article copies available for a fee from The Haworth Document Delivery Service: 1-800-HAWORTH. E-mail address: <docdelivery@haworthpress.com>*

David W. Coon, PhD, is affiliated with the Department of Social & Behavioral Sciences, Arizona State University, MC 3051, 4701 W. Thunderbird Rd., Glendale, AZ 85306-4908 (E-mail: david.w.coon@asu.edu).

[Haworth co-indexing entry note]: "Exploring Interventions for LGBT Caregivers: Issues and Examples." Coon, David W. Co-published simultaneously in *Journal of Gay & Lesbian Social Services* (The Haworth Press, Inc.) Vol. 18, No. 3/4, 2007, pp. 109-128; and: *Caregiving with Pride* (ed: Karen I. Fredriksen-Goldsen) The Haworth Press, Inc., 2007, pp. 109-128. Single or multiple copies of this article are available for a fee from The Haworth Document Delivery Service [1-800-HAWORTH, 9:00 a.m. - 5:00 p.m. (EST). E-mail address: docdelivery@haworthpress.com].

KEYWORDS. Caregiving, intervention, lesbian, gay, bisexual, transgender, LGBT, older adults, aging, SURE 2

I know how lucky I am. My parents and siblings in rural [America] love Todd [his partner of over 20 years]. My younger brother and sister-in-law drove out last year and we traveled to the coast together; them helping me watch out for Todd. . . . Of course, there were a few stressed moments. But, just like our gay and lesbian friends like Jill and Pat, they haven't abandoned us. Can't say that about everyone, of course . . . but I am lucky. (Coon & Zeiss, 2003b, p. 269)

We often talk about that book [Kath Weston's *Families We Choose: Lesbians, Gays, Kinship*]. My family is really both: it's my nuclear, my blood family and it's the gay and lesbian family Todd and I chose together here in the city and from back home, years ago. Many of them are still with us. They are our champions. (Coon & Zeiss, 2003b, p. 289)

THE NEED FOR TARGETED CAREGIVER INTERVENTIONS IN THE LGBT COMMUNITY

Clearly, as the quotations above remind us, lesbian, gay, bisexual and transgender (LGBT) caregivers can receive support from LGBT family and friends, as well as biological family members and friends from the larger heterosexual community (i.e., "the majority"). Therefore, one must avoid the stereotype of LGBT caregivers and care recipients as solely disowned and isolated from informal and formal social support systems designed to support majority caregivers. However, until LGBT caregivers no longer face the discrimination that builds barriers to competent care for their care recipients or that heightens impediments to programs and services needed to sustain LGBT caregivers in their role, this article takes the position found in earlier work (e.g., Coon & Burleson, 2006): Ethical standards demand that professionals, regardless of sexual orientation, expand their understanding of LGBT caregiving issues and deepen their competence in provision of LGBT caregiver referrals and services.

The Impact of Caregiving

LGBT service providers unfamiliar with caregiving issues may question the need for LGBT caregiver services, given the budgetary challenges many LGBT community based organizations face today. However, caregiving for a partner, relative or friend comes with numerous tasks and burdens that can frequently change across the course of an illness or disability. As a result, caregivers have often been referred to as hidden patients (Fengler & Goodrich, 1979), because the need to balance the caregiving role and its changing responsibilities with other important social roles (e.g., employee, partner, volunteer, parent, or friend) can yield substantial levels of stress and distress. While most informal caregivers report elevated levels of stress and distress (Administration on Aging, 2000; Bookwala, Yee, & Schulz, 2000; Schulz, O'Brien, Bookwala, & Fleissner, 1995), some caregiving roles, most notably the role of dementia caregiver, can lead to significantly higher levels of psychological, physical, social and economic burden and related distress (Ory, Hoffman, Yee, Tennstedt, & Schulz, 1999). Moreover, recent caregiver research has demonstrated that caregiver stress, if left unchecked, can place caregivers at higher risk for mortality, identifying a serious public health issue. More specifically, older adults who experienced strain in the role of caring for a disabled spouse in this study were 63% more likely to die within 4 years than noncaregivers (Schulz & Beach, 1999).

LGBT Caregiving Related Surveys

Unfortunately, the face of the LGBT caregiver has been missing from much of the scientific research on informal caregiving. Although many of the accounts to date that explore LGBT caregiving appear in the HIV/AIDS literature (e.g., Fredriksen, 1999; Wight, 2002), results from several surveys with LGBT older adults and caregivers in larger US cities (i.e., New York, San Francisco, San Jose) are beginning to emerge (Cantor, Brennan, & Shippy, 2004; Hoctel, 2002; Outword Online, 2000). These surveys are helping to provide valid data on LGBT caregivers to older adults. For example, similar to smaller LGBT caregiver surveys, a recent survey of 341 LGBT New Yorkers age 50 and older found that older LGBT individuals serve as caregivers for aging parents and other dependent biological family members, as well as partners and friends (Cantor et al., 2004). In general, they provide help to care recipients in ways very similar to heterosexual caregivers, including hands-on assistance, "care management" activities (e.g., arranging home care), and emotional support. However, the survey also found that one third of almost 350 LGBT older adults reported biological family members expected more caregiving responsibilities of them because they were LGBT and "single," making the assumption that they had fewer explicit family responsibilities. This assumption typically was found to be false (Cantor et al., 2004), demonstrating that biological family members can frequently ignore LGBT primary partnerships or nontraditional family relationships.

In contrast to their heterosexual counterparts, findings from several of these surveys also suggest that LGBT caregivers and older adults experience a good deal of discrimination that discourages self-disclosure and creates barriers to service utilization. For example, in a recent San Francisco survey of approximately 50 LGBT caregivers and 50 LGBT individuals concerned about their current or near future care needs, 35.2% of caregivers and 54.8% of care recipients reported they would not seek outside help because of perceived barriers related to sexual orientation (e.g., concerns about harassment and provider lack of sensitivity) (Coon & Zeiss, 2003a). Notably, many of the issues described in this article are drawn from experience and data gathered from LGBT caregivers and helping professionals in cities like San Francisco, New York City, and Los Angeles, cities that have larger, more visible LGBT communities. Concerned providers and interested researchers may ask "What do LGBT caregivers and care recipients experience living in places without an established community?" Unfortunately, while this data remains unavailable, barriers to LGBT caregiver service utilization in smaller cities and rural areas may only be intensified by fewer LGBT friendly resources and greater social isolation (Coon & Zeiss, 2003b).

Considering Caregiver Sociocultural Contexts

The sociocultural context can significantly shape LBGT caregiver beliefs about and responses to illness and disability, perceptions of caregiver stress and distress, and the acceptability of help-seeking behavior and service utilization (Gallagher-Thompson, Hargrave, et al., 2003). Today's LGBT caregivers encompass a diverse group in terms of ethnicity, race, language, national origin, and physical challenges and often crisscross a variety of these cohort and sociocultural boundaries. As a result, many LGBT caregivers may face double, triple or quadruple forms of jeopardy when they hold other minority status (Greene, 1994). In addition, LGBT caregivers, because of their relationships, roles and responsibilities, often sit at the intersection of topics of key concern to the LGBT community including gay marriage, the limitations of domestic partner benefits such as lack of tax benefits and decision-making power automatically given to biological relatives when impaired, and the impact of discrimination in the Family and Medical Leave Act.

LGBT caregivers include not only those caring for family of origin members (e.g., parents and siblings), but also individuals caring for people representing their families of choice (e.g., partners, neighbors, and friends). Still, professionals must remember that it is predominantly the "out" group of caregivers who self-identify as LGBT that are more likely to access LGBT specific support services. Other LGBT caregivers, depending upon their level of outness, may remain more reticent with healthcare and social service providers, and consequently not self-identify to be "counted" in intake forms, surveys or questionnaires. This may be especially the case for older LGBT cohorts who faced multiple years of discrimination and intolerance, and may now have those feelings intensified by other forms of discrimination (e.g., ageism, sexism, racism, or discrimination based on disabilities) (Barón & Cramer, 2000). For example, about 25% of recent respondents to a New York LGBT older adult survey said they were open to no one and over 50% did not completely disclose their sexual orientation to their health care providers (Cantor et al., 2004), an issue that can easily impact quality of care and informal caregiving.

Professionals involved in either LGBT identified or caregiver targeted programs and services must consider that several aspects of the sociocultural context impact LGBT caregivers and their care recipients in distinctly different ways than their heterosexual peers. These include issues related to cultural, historical, employment, financial, legal, informal support and spiritual contexts (for additional information, see Cahill, South, & Spade, 2000; Coon & Burleson, 2006; Coon & Zeiss, 2003b). For example, cultural proscriptions vary in their openness about sexuality and the ramifications of violating prohibitions (e.g., Choi, Salazar, Lew, & Coates, 1995; Fukuyama & Ferguson, 2000; Moore, 1997; Ross, Paulsen, & Stalstrom, 1988), thereby influencing whether or not information is altered or withheld or more anonymous caregiver services are preferred to protect one's identity. In a relatively short historical period, the sociocultural environment has changed quite drastically for many midlife and older LGBT cohorts. These cohorts may have legitimate uneasiness about how well service providers understand their particular contexts and concerns, which often differ substantively from those of younger cohorts (Kimmel, 1995). Recent work with 416 LGB older adults aged 60 or older indicated that nearly 75%

reported some kind of sexual orientation victimization, with men reporting more overall victimization than women. The impact of this victimization is telling: Participants who had been physically attacked reported poorer mental health outcomes including more suicide attempts than other participants (D'Augelli & Grossman, 2001). Thus, given these negative experiences, older LGBT caregivers may hold extremely mixed feelings about openly seeking help (Coon & Zeiss, 2003).

In terms of employment, legal and financial contexts, numerous privileges taken for granted by heterosexuals are often difficult to obtain or flatly denied to LGBT caregivers. While caregiving often negatively impacts caregiver employment regardless of sexual orientation (Ory et al., 1999), these issues are quickly compounded among LGBT caregivers when being "out" at work can result in both economic and psychosocial stressors based on both overt and covert discrimination (e.g., Alexander, 1997; Croteau, Anderson, Distefano, & Kampa-Kokesch, 2000). LGBT individuals may also face barriers to health care coverage, since they are ineligible for benefits typically extended to legally married spouses, and are typically discriminated against, no matter the length of their partnership, in terms of survival benefits, inheritance rights, and community property rights.

The informal social support context often plays a unique role in helping buffer caregivers from the responsibilities and stresses of regular care. From the outset, service providers need to avoid the stereotype that all older LGBT persons do not have children or are inevitably alone. Recent research with New York LGBT caregivers suggests that LGBT caregiver support networks encompass a variety of family of origin relationships with the vast majority feeling at least somewhat if not very close to these network members. For example, approximately 33% had living parents, 75% had siblings, and 20% had children. In terms of network members from their family of choice, 40% of the New York respondents were partnered, and over 90% reported an average of six friends, with 96% stating they felt somewhat or very close to friends (Cantor et al., 2004). Still, the type of support LGBT caregivers need remains unclear and may be quite individualistic since LGBT individuals, in contrast to older heterosexuals, may have let go of unrealistic expectations that blood relatives or friends will provide for them beyond a certain point (Quam & Whitford, 1992). LGBT caregivers also may have let go of rigid sex roles or divisions of labor that may increase their willingness to do tasks once managed by ailing partners. Finally, professionals need to consider that future cohorts of caregiving gay men severely impacted by the HIV/AIDS epidemic may have more attenuated informal networks upon which to rely (Coon, 2003).

Religious coping is a frequently used, if not the most frequently used, type of coping reported by caregivers (e.g., NAC/AARP, 2004). However, even though some religious organizations are reexamining, or have made changes in, their views on homosexuality, few religious organizations still truly welcome "out" LGBT individuals. Thus, today's LGBT caregivers and care recipients looking to incorporate religious or spiritual coping into their lives often struggle in their attempts to uphold, adapt or discard religious doctrine and spiritual beliefs discordant with their sexual orientation (Kellems & Fassinger, 2003). While many LGBT caregivers may not feel that they can turn to religious or spiritual coping based in the religion of their youth, the heterogeneity within the LGBT community suggests that others may find their religious communities and spiritual beliefs to be of immense importance in coping with life stressors such as caregiving struggles. For example, about 20% of the New York LGBT caregivers surveyed stated that they had turned to clergy for advice and support (Cantor et al., 2004). This may be particularly true for LGBT persons of color where religion and spirituality remain a refuge against racial and ethnic discrimination (e.g., Davidson, 2000; Fukuyama & Ferguson, 2000).

Need for Multiple Levels of Intervention

In addition to the various obstacles that arose in consideration of the caregiver's sociocultural contexts, obstacles can be found across multiple levels of service provision and intervention. These obstacles can range from impediments at the individual or interpersonal levels of behavior change as well as barriers to proactive organizational or system levels of change all the way up to roadblocks forstalling initiatives designed to positively transform communities and shape influential policy. Yet, one common theme–that of hatred, discrimination and intolerance (DiPlacido, 1998; Herek, Gillis, & Cogan, 1999)–weaves itself throughout these levels negatively impacting LGBT caregivers and their service providers. For example, service providers must consider at the individual or interpersonal level that the two individuals in an LGBT caregiver-care recipient dyad may be differentially "out" and now may be forced "out" or "in" to obtain needed services, thereby exacerbating stress and distress. Reports of discrimination after disclosure of sexual orientation in service provision like health care providers and senior centers (e.g., Dean et al., 2002; Kauth, Harwig & Kalichman, 2000;

Wolfe, 2000) are particularly disturbing for those trying to reach out to and effectively serve LGBT caregivers and care recipients. Organizations at the system level of service provision can automatically hand decision making power to biological relatives rather than longtime partners, refuse LGBT partners visitation rights, openly discriminate against LGBT applicants in long term care, and ignore LGBT issues in staff diversity training.

The sociocultural contexts discussed earlier also can raise awareness about obstacles at the community level, ranging from particular geographic regions or municipalities with minimal protection for LGBT persons to communities based on religious faith that actively drive out LGBT members. Unfortunately, the LGBT community itself, or at least certain segments of the community, may hold prejudices that place LGBT caregivers and care recipients at risk. For example, ageism may be reflected in the limited availability of formal support systems for LGBT older adults and their caregivers, even in well-established LGBT communities (Coon & Zeiss, 2003; Grossman et al., 2000). Additional policy level barriers range from lack of domestic partner benefits, including spousal benefits, disability benefits, and retirement benefits for same sex partners, to lack of anti-discrimination policies protecting employment, public housing, and access and delivery of services based on sexual orientation (Cahill et al., 2000). For example, many LGBT older adults have been partnered for decades, but without recognition of same-sex marriages or civil unions, they cannot benefit from recognition by governmental entities and public policy frameworks that married heterosexual couples rely upon, including tax benefits (Cantor et al., 2004). As a result, same sex couples cannot accrue as much savings and have fewer financial resources in later life that directly impact the kind of caregiving assistance they can afford.

The multiple levels of obstacles faced by LGBT caregivers and care recipients uncover the need for multiple levels of complementary intervention. At the individual or interpersonal level, organizations could create and support both face-to-face and online LGBT caregiver and care recipient support groups. LGBT community-based organizations, senior service organizations, health care organizations, and local area agencies on aging could form partnerships and pool resources at the system or organizational level of intervention to design and implement effective care pathways for LGBT caregivers and care recipients. As an example of interventions targeted at the community level, newly forming LGBT retirement communities could be encouraged to incorporate community education and training to help inform the entire retirement community about caregiving and provide booster training programs as needed. Continuing to champion the National Family Caregiver Support program's broad definition of "family" to help support those providing care to LGBT older adults could serve as an example of one way to intervene at the policy intervention level. Readers interested in addition information and examples of strategies to overcome barriers to LGBT caregiver service provision and utilization are referred to Cahill and colleagues (2000), Coon (2003), and Coon and Burleson (2006).

SURE 2 FRAMEWORK WITH LGBT CAREGIVERS

The SURE 2 framework was developed in response to the multiple levels of service utilization barriers LGBT caregivers face while trying to find support for their care recipients and address their own caregiving concerns. Targeted at the individual/interpersonal intervention level, SURE 2 acknowledges that while LGBT caregivers may share many of the same concerns as heterosexual caregivers, such as acceptance of a disease process or disability, grief and loss issues, and conflicts with informal and formal support systems, SURE 2 also recognizes that LGBT caregivers identify and share concerns that appear specific to them and their situations (Coon & Zeiss, 2003b; Levine & Altman, 2002). For example, many LGBT caregivers seek provider assistance to more effectively manage one or more of the following: (a) differences between themselves and their emerging or possible selves (e.g., coming out of the closet to family or employers to help them manage their caregiving situation or coming out as a caregiver through revealing their loved one's emergent illness or disability); (b) issues pertaining to significant others including the care recipient, family of origin and family of choice whose own internalized homophobia and ageism may add yet another stressor to already overwhelmed caregivers (e.g., some LGBT caregivers may now be caring for a family member who shunned them for decades because of their sexual orientation or gender identity); and, (c) conflicts or tensions between themselves and their "communities" (e.g., struggling with the limited attention by the LGBT community to its older members and caregiving issues, and the heterosexist attitudes and policies of other communities that negatively impact LGBT caregivers' physical, emotional, spiritual and social quality of life).

Blending key elements of grass roots support groups with basic cognitive and behavioral skill-building techniques (CBT) (e.g., Beck, Rush, Shaw & Emery, 1979; Lewinsohn, Muñoz, Youngren, & Zeiss, 1986), the SURE 2 model provides a simple framework that providers and administrators can easily adapt for a variety of situations and settings (Coon & Zeiss, 2003b). For example, while SURE 2 was developed for an open ended two–hour, monthly LGBT dementia caregiver support group in San Francisco, it can be extended to time-limited interventions or to caregivers of patients with other types of illnesses. The framework has been applied successfully in individual, couple and family counseling, but could easily be adapted for other individual or interpersonal levels of intervention such as individual, couple or family care management and consultation, or more focused psychoeducational skill-building groups that target both the caregiver and the care recipient.

Perspective, Goals and Outcomes

Grounded in an empowerment perspective that encourages LGBT caregivers to empower one another and themselves through support, education, skill development, and active engagement,, the SURE 2 model consists of 2 S's (Sharing & Support), U's (Unhelpful Thoughts/Behaviors & Understanding), R's (Reframes & Referrals), and E's (Education & Exploration). The acronym is intended to be simple for facilitators/interventionists to remember, to introduce and review when needed, and to build upon and reinforce when presented with LGBT caregivers in a variety of settings and situations.

One overarching goal of the SURE2 framework is the recognition of the sociocultural context raised earlier, a context within which caregivers live and function. The sociocultural context creates common ground that is shared or at least understood by most LGBT caregivers and also recognizes unique features of the sociocultural landscape individualized to a particular caregiver or group of caregivers. For example, cultural minority groups, in contrast to non-Hispanic Whites in the LGBT community, often have had to face multiple forms of discrimination, including a lack of acceptance within the predominantly White organized LGBT community. Thus, the SURE2 framework acknowledges that the provision of a "safe place" (Coon & Zeiss, 2003b) is critical in the development of successful interventions for LGBT caregivers. Caregivers need a place in which LGBT individuals can discuss their roles as caregivers in tandem with other roles ranging from partner, friend, and family member to employee, citizen and volunteer, while at the same time openly expressing the challenges that can emerge in balancing an LGBT sexual orientation or identity with this caregiving role in hostile or dismissive sociocultural contexts.

The SURE 2 framework also emphasizes the development of proximal goals closely tied to key caregiver outcomes, including the lessening of stress and distress, the enhancement of positive coping strategies and the reduction of negative coping strategies, and the increase in social support satisfaction. These goals and outcomes are to be achieved through education, support, and the development and practice of skills based in cognitive behavioral theories of mood management (Beck et al., 1979; Lewinsohn et al., 1986). Goals and outcomes are further supported through the identification and use of LGBT sensitive and "caregiving competent" formal service provider referrals. Moreover, SURE 2 incorporates the construct of self-efficacy (Bandura, 1997), positing that caregiver self-efficacy beliefs or the confidence one has in their ability to carry out various aspects of their caregiving role influences the initiation of actions. Therefore, self-efficacy serves as an important mediator of behavior not only in caregiving, but also in other life roles. As such, the development of LGBT caregiver self-efficacy becomes an important mechanism of change, and another key goal, providing the mechanism through which the SURE 2 intervention is to accomplish its other goals and achieve its key outcomes.

The SURE 2 framework was designed to be delivered by well trained providers or well trained and supervised volunteers who can effectively utilize the SURE 2 components to create the opportunity for honest open communication regarding caregiver stress and LGBT-specific concerns. Those trained in the SURE 2 framework, in turn, can use its components to help caregivers develop the skills to move from viewing their situations as primarily consisting of overwhelming challenges and related distress to being able to see a set of more manageable problems and finding ways to reduce their stress while maintaining their caregiving role (Coon & Zeiss, 2003b).

SURE 2 Components

In brief, SURE 2 caregivers are encouraged to reframe their thinking and change their behavior through basic problem-solving, positive reframing and other CBT techniques, and to elicit ideas from the group. These approaches are based on successful interventions appearing in the research literature that were tested through randomized clinical trials (Coon et al., 2003; Gallagher-Thompson et al., 2003; REACH II Investigators, in press). However, SURE 2, in contrast to these other interventions, specifically creates a safe place for LGBT caregivers to identify unique obstacles they face, such as the challenges of managing "outness" effectively, handling hostile biological relatives, and finding LGBT-sensitive services. SURE 2's key components include the following.

Sharing and Support. SURE 2, in the tradition of many grass roots support groups, clearly affords time for group members to share their feelings regarding caregiving and its impact on their emotional, physical, social and financial health. However, in terms of structure, the groups are organized into two distinct yet interrelated phases. Each group meeting begins with a traditional introduction and check-in where caregivers not only introduce themselves, but also place items on the table they would like to examine more fully. Introductions occur at the first meeting of each closed or time-limited groups or at each meeting in open ended groups where subsequent meetings may draw new participants. "Crosstalk" during check in is limited to clarifying questions to increase group understanding of the basic issue to be placed on the table. The focus on informational and emotional support emerges after check-in when those items on the table are discussed more fully. The facilitator in cooperation with group members prioritizes discussion items, often grouping issues together by drawing relationships among participant concerns and then working together to identify the most pressing concerns to discuss first. This process yields a natural agenda that helps the group transition from check in to the next phase of the meeting. The remainder of the meeting blends sharing and support with other components that emphasize education, skill development, and appropriate referrals.

Unhelpful Thoughts/Behaviors and *Understanding.* While sharing and support provide a solid foundation for SURE 2 groups, the framework also builds upon psychoeducational skill development perspectives that integrate basic CBT principles. These perspectives suggest that for groups to be most effective, facilitators need to help caregivers maximize their effective coping skills as well as learn and try out new skills and strategies demonstrated by other participants and/or the facilitator (Thompson, Powers, Coon, Takagi, McKibbin, & Gallagher-Thompson, 2000).

The first step in this process involves helping group members identify unhelpful thinking and behavior patterns that negatively impact their emotional, physical and social health. Identification occurs through the discussion of the conflicts, stressors, or issues placed on the table during check in, whether it be a conflict between caregivers and significant others including the care recipients, frustrations with health care systems, legal challenges, or any other issue. In any case, the group encourages participants facing the issue under discussion to identify what is and is not working in their attempts to cope and manage the situation. Group members, in turn, share their empathy and understanding of how easy it is to get caught up in negative thinking about themselves, others, and the future. Similarly, the facilitator and other group members learn to recognize and acknowledge how frequently caregivers do not take care of themselves when trying to balance caregiving and other responsibilities, and how often instead caregivers reach for unhelpful behaviors, such as worrying, eating, drinking, smoking, or working too much in their attempts to manage daily stressors. Thus, the group on the one hand helps normalize the process of reaching for unhelpful thinking and behavioral strategies, while on the other emphasizing the importance of developing new and implementing existing skills that are more likely to reduce stress, alleviate emotional distress and enhance coping.

Reframes and *Referrals.* SURE 2 group members are urged to move beyond just the identification of negative patterns of thought and action and the expressions of support and understanding regarding the issues faced by fellow members. Rather, SURE 2 functions in some ways as an education and training site where participants are encouraged to consider ways to reframe their thinking and change their behavior through basic cognitive restructuring techniques (e.g., basic problem solving, cost/benefit analyses, avoiding black and white thinking and positive re-framing) and behavioral strategies (assertive communication skills, time management and pleasant events scheduling) and by eliciting ideas and perspectives from the group. These ideas also include recognition of the obstacles LGBT people face as a result of their sexual orientation or identity, such as difficulty finding LGBT sensitive in home health care, day care or appropriate placement situations, the challenges of managing "outness" effectively across multiple domains (e.g., family, friends, neighbors, employers, health care and social service providers, and religious leaders and congregations), and the additional financial and legal planning burdens that results from the lack of formal recognition of LGBT partnerships. The facilitator and group members share appropriate referrals when competent professionals and organizations have been identified to help overcome some of these obstacles. Unmistakably, many group members come to the group with at least some healthy coping strategies that already work for them, and the group process is used in such instances to help acknowledge, reinforce and sustain the use of these strategies.

Education and *Exploration.* SURE 2 includes basic education about the care recipient's disease and issues regarding co-morbidities, as well as caregiver-related information such as information regarding the course of caregiving. Depending on the format of the group, expert speakers may be invited for brief presentations followed by a question and answer period (total combined time of 30-45 minutes). Experts speak and answer questions at the beginning of the group, allowing 75 to 90 minutes after they leave for member check in followed by the usual group discussion designed to address issues raised during check in. Education also includes facilitator and group identification of upcoming educational seminars relevant to members such as those sponsored by local chapters of the Alzheimer's Association. It may include a brief overview of recent research findings relevant to the group, or occasionally a quick discussion regarding research opportunities in the area. In this educational role, SURE 2 can help members become more informed consumers of research by brainstorming key questions caregivers would want answered about a research opportunity prior to becoming involved or additional information they would want to help them better understand research findings in the press. Voluntary health organizations (e.g., Alzheimer's Association or the American Cancer Society) may have printed and/or web-based press releases or summaries of recent research findings that can be mentioned or given to participants as appropriate.

Each SURE 2 encounter also allows time at the end to explore caregiver experiences with key strategies that have not already been covered during open discussion using Reframes and Referrals. These typically include recent explorations by group members of alternative coping strategies or community referrals that members tried. What did or did not work, and why? During this time, caregivers can provide feedback to one another about their experience with coping alternatives and recent referrals, including the referral's understanding of not only caregiving situations but also their sensitivity to issues faced by LGBT caregivers. This process brings to the forefront whether or not programs and services are available, accessible, and acceptable to LGBT caregivers. The general assumption is the focus will be on the lack of caregiving programs and services that are LGBT sensitive with competent professionals who can help LGBT caregivers manage their caregiving responsibilities and related stress. Indeed this is frequently the case; however, one quickly learns that LGBT services often are not "caregiving competent" as well, and lack professionals who understand the unique challenges LGBT caregivers face. Finally, SURE 2 groups close with an exploration of at least one cognitive or behavioral strategy and at least one referral (when appropriate) for each caregiver to try before the next meeting. Since caregivers often focus on strategies to assist the care recipient, this last round of exploration specifically focus on strategies and referrals designed to help them take care of themselves in the course of their caregiving careers.

A LOOK TOWARD THE FUTURE

After decades of caregiver intervention design, implementation and evaluation, no one best intervention has been identified for caregivers to ill or disabled midlife and older adults (Bourgeois, Schulz & Burgio, 1996; Gallagher-Thompson & Coon, in press; Kennet, Burgio, & Schulz, 2000). In part, this may be due not only to the multiple levels of obstacles family caregivers face in today's world, but also to the diversity of today's caregivers, including the different sociocultural contexts within which they live and provide care. Similarly, the diversity of the LGBT community and the additional obstacles LGBT caregivers face suggests that no single "one size fits all" intervention will meet the needs of all the community's caregivers.

However, several key findings have emerged from the scientific literature that may prove useful in the development of interventions for LGBT caregivers, particularly with regard to interventions targeted at the individual or interpersonal level. These research results suggest that interventions designed to help caregivers develop skills to reduce their own stress levels and manage care recipient behavior problems can be effective in alleviating caregiver distress (e.g., Buckwalter, Gernder, Kohout, & Hall, 1999; Gallagher-Thompson et al., 2003; Teri, Logsdon, Uomoto & McCurry, 1997). The power of these skill-based intervention strategies appears to be further enhanced when they are individually tailored to meet caregiver needs and combined with other aspects of education, support and counseling (e.g., Mittelman, Roth, Coon & Healy, 2004; REACH II Investigators, in press). Moreover, other promising approaches are also arriving on the caregiver intervention scene. Technological approaches such as telephone-based technologies or online support combined with skill-focused education (e.g., Eisdorfer et al., 2003; Steffen) and modifications of the physical environments of the caregiving dyad to help support its functioning (Gitlin et al., 2003) may also be effective.

The SURE 2 framework is one example of a LGBT caregiver intervention that builds on many of the principles found in the scientific literature. SURE 2, although directed at the individual/interpersonal intervention level, is also designed to help LGBT caregivers identify and share information that impacts stressors experienced at other levels of service provision and intervention, and uses CBT-based techniques to develop skills to help caregivers manage stress. While SURE 2 was developed for dementia caregivers and used with caregivers to midlife and older adults with chronic illness or disability, many of its components can be easily adapted for or extended to other types of caregivers. Unfortunately, no randomized clinical trials of successful intervention approaches have been extended specifically to LGBT caregivers. However, the time has come and the SURE 2 model could be evaluated in this way. SURE 2 would also benefit from more fully developed training manuals that would be needed for experimental research.

The SURE 2 model could also be extended to other caregivers technologically, that is, through telephone or online interaction. In this way, SURE 2 could reach closeted LGBT caregivers who want a level of anonymity, and/or LGBT caregivers "confined" at home due to transportation barriers or as a result of their caregiving duties, allowing them to connect with others. It might also be a mechanism by which those living in rural areas or other areas without a well-defined LGBT community learn from one another. Although many of the successful interventions identified in the scientific literature may be more intensive and, therefore, more costly than many service organizations can afford to deliver, such technological approaches may actually allow organizations to share costs with programs serving other populations (e.g., LGBT youth or shut-ins).

The LGBT community and its caregivers and care recipients might also benefit from intergenerational or multigenerational intervention approaches that combine education, support and skills-based training to alleviate caregiver distress, to enhance care recipient quality of life, and to strengthen the social compact. The discussion herein has focused on the challenges encountered by LGBT caregivers; however, heterosexual and LGBT caregivers alike are often able to describe positive aspects of caregiving that support them in their caregiving journey (Cantor et al., 2004; Roth et al., 2004). These positive aspects or caregiver gains point to other opportunities for intervention design and development grounded in strength-based approaches. Finally, practitioners and clinical researchers must remain mindful that given the array of obstacles faced by many LGBT caregivers, future LGBT caregiver interventions must identify strategies that help caregivers successfully overcome these obstacles, and subsequently create purposeful linkages among effective interventions developed at each level (Coon & Burleson, 2006; Emmons, 2001).

REFERENCES

Administration on Aging. (2000). America's families care: A report on the needs of America's family caregivers. Retrieved from: http://www.aoa.dhhs.gov/carenetwork/report.html

Alexander, C. J. (1997). *Growth and intimacy for gay men*. New York: Harrington Park Press.

Bandura, A. (1997). *Self-efficacy: The exercise of control*. New York: W.H. Freeman & Co.

Barón, A., & Cramer, D. (2000). Potential counseling concerns of aging lesbian, gay, and bisexual clients. In, R.M. Perez, K.A. DeBord, K.J. Bieschke, *Handbook of counseling and psychotherapy with lesbian, gay, and bisexual clients* (pp. 207-224). Washington, D.C.: American Psychological Association.

Beck, A. T., Rush, A. J., Shaw, B. F., & Emery, G. (1979). *Cognitive therapy of depression*. New York: Guilford Press.

Bookwala, J., Yee, J. L., & Schulz, R. (2000). Caregiving and detrimental mental and physical health outcomes. In G. M. Williamson, P. A. Parmelee, & D. R. Shaffer (Eds.), *Physical illness and depression in older adults: A handbook of theory, research, and practice* (pp. 93-131). New York: Plenum.

Bourgeois, M. S., Schulz, R., & Burgio, L. (1996). Intervention for caregivers of patients with Alzheimer's disease: A review and analysis of content, process, and outcomes. *International Journal of Human Development, 43*, 35-92.

Buckwalter, K., C., Gerdner, L., Kohout, F., Richards-Hall, G., Kelly, A., Richards, B., & Sime, M. (1999). A nursing intervention to decrease depression in family caregivers of persons with dementia. *Archives of Psychiatric Nursing, 13*, 80-88.

Cahill, S., South, K., & Spade, J. (2000). *Outing age: Public policy issues affecting gay, lesbian, bisexual and transgender elders*. New York: The Policy Institute of the National Gay and Lesbian Task Force Foundation. Available at www.ngltf.org

Cantor, M. H., Brennan, M., & Shippy, R. A. (2004). *Caregiving among older lesbian, gay, bisexual and transgender New Yorkers*. New York: National Gay and Lesbian Task Force Policy Institute.

Choi, K. H., Salazar, N., Lew, S., & Coates, T. J. (1995). In B. Greene, & Herek, G. M. (Eds.), *Psychological perspectives on lesbian and gay issues: Vol. 2. AIDS identity and community: The HIV epidemic and lesbians and gay men*. Thousand Oaks, CA: Sage.

Coon, D. W. (2003). *Lesbian, gay, bisexual and transgender (LGBT) issues and family caregiving*. The National Center on Caregiving, Family Caregiver Alliance, San Francisco, CA.

Coon, D. W. & Burleson, M. H. (2006). Working with gay, lesbian, bisexual, and transgender families. In Yeo, G. & Gallagher-Thompson, D. (Eds.) *Ethnicity & the dementias* (2nd ed.) (pp. 343-358). New York: Routledge Taylor & Francis Group.

Coon, D. W., Thompson, L. W., Steffen. A., Sorocco, K., & Gallagher-Thompson, D. (2003). Anger and depression management: Psychoeducational skill training interventions for women caregivers of a relative with dementia. *The Gerontologist, 43,* 678-689.

Coon, D. W., & Zeiss, L. M. (2003a). Caring for families we choose: Intervention issues with LGBT caregivers. In D. W. Coon, *Dementia caregiving interventions: Intersections of gender, sexual orientation and culture.* Symposium presented at the National Multicultural Conference and Summit III, Los Angeles, CA.

Coon, D. W., & Zeiss, L. M. (2003b). The families we choose: Intervention issues with LGBT caregivers. In Coon, D. W., Gallagher-Thompson, D. & Thompson, L. (Eds.). *Innovative interventions to reduce dementia caregiver distress: A clinical guide* (pp. 267-295). New York: Springer.

Croteau, J. M., Anderson, M. Z., Distefano, T. M., & Kampa-Kokesch, S. (2000). In. R. Perez, K. A. DeBord, & K. J Bieschke, (Eds.), *Handbook of counseling and psychotherapy with lesbian, gay, and bisexual clients.* Washington, D.C.: American Psychological Association.

D'Augelli, A. R & Grossman, A. H. (2001). Disclosure of sexual orientation, victimization, and mental health among lesbian, gay and bisexual older adults. *Journal of Interpersonal Violence, 16,* 1008-1027.

Davidson, M. G. (2000). Religion and spirituality. In R. Perez, K. A. DeBord, & K. J. Bieschke, (Eds.). *Handbook of counseling and psychotherapy with lesbian, gay, and bisexual clients* (pp. 409-434). Washington, D.C.: American Psychological Association.

Dean, L., Meyer, I. H., Robinson, K., Sell, R. L., Sember, R., Silenzio, V. M. B., et al., (2000, October). Lesbian, gay, bisexual and transgender health: Findings and concerns. *Journal of the Gay and Lesbian Medical Association, 4,* 101-151. Available free online at http://www.glma.org/pub/jglma/index.shtml

DiPlacido, J. (1998). Minority stress among lesbians, gay men, and bisexuals: A consequence of heterosexism, homophobia, and stigmatization. In G. Herek (Ed.), Psychological perspectives on lesbian and gay issues: Vol. 4. Stigma and sexual orientation: *Understanding prejudice against lesbians, gay men, and bisexuals* (pp. 138-159). Thousand Oaks, CA: Sage.

Eisdorfer, C., Czaja, S. J., Loewenstein, D. A., Rubert, M. P., Argüelles, S., Mitrani, V. B., Szapocznik, J. (2003). The effect of a family therapy and technology-based intervention on caregiver depression. *The Gerontologist, 43,* 521-531.

Emmons, K. M. (2001). Behavioral and social science contributions to the health of adults in the United States. In B. D. Smedley & S. L. Syme (Ed.), *Promoting health: Intervention strategies from social and behavioral research,* (pp. 254-321). Washington, DC: National Academy Press.

Fengler, A. P., & Goodrich, N. (1979). Wives of elderly disabled men: The hidden patients. *The Gerontologist, 19,* 175-183.

Fredriksen, K. L. (1999). Family caregiving responsibilities among lesbians and gay men. *Social Work, 44,* 142-155.

Fukuyama, M. A., & Ferguson, A. D. (2000). Lesbian, gay, and bisexual people of color: Understanding cultural complexity and managing multiple oppressions. In R. Perez, K. A DeBord, & K. J. Bieschke, (Eds.) *Handbook of counseling and psychotherapy with lesbian, gay, and bisexual clients.* Washington, D.C.: American Psychological Association.

Gallagher-Thompson, D., & Coon, D. W. (in press). Evidence-based treatments to reduce psychological distress in family caregivers of older adults. *Psychology & Aging.*

Gallagher-Thompson, D., Coon, D., Solano, N., Ambler, C., Rabinowitz, R. & Thompson, L. (2003). Change in indices of distress among Latina and Anglo female caregivers of elderly relatives with dementia: Site specific results from the REACH National Collaborative Study. *The Gerontologist, 43,* 580-591.

Gallagher-Thompson, D., Hargrave, R., Hinton, L., Arean, P., Iwamasa, G., & Zeiss, L. M. (2003). Interventions for a multicultural society. In D. Coon, D. Gallagher-Thompson, & L. W. Thompson (Eds.), *Innovative interventions to reduce dementia caregiver distress: A clinical guide* (pp. 50-73). New York: Springer.

Gitlin, L. N., Winter, L., Corcoran, M., Dennis, M., Schinfeld, S., & Hauck, W. (2003). Effects of the Home Environmental Skill-building Program on the Caregiver-Care Recipient Dyad: Six-month Outcomes from the Philadelphia REACH Initiative. *The Gerontologist, 43,* 532-546.

Greene, B. (1994). Ethnic minority lesbians and gay men: Mental health and treatment issues. *Journal of Consulting and Clinical Psychology, 62,* 243 251.

Grossman, A. H., D'Augelli, A. R., Hershberger, S. L. (2000). Social support networks of lesbian, gay, and bisexual adults 60 years of age and older. *Journal of Gerontology, 55B,* P171-P179.

Herek, G. M., Gillis, J. R., & Cogan, J. C. (1999). Psychological sequelae of hate crime victimization among lesbian, gay, and bisexual adults. *Journal of Consulting and Clinical Psychology, 67,* 945-951.

Hoctel, P. D. (2002, January-February). Community assessments show service gaps for LGBT elders. *Aging Today, 23,* 5-6.

Kauth, M. R., Hartwig, M. J., & Kalichman, S. C. (2000). Health behavior relevant to psychotherapy with lesbian, gay, and bisexual clients. In R. Perez, K. A. DeBord, & K. J.Bieschke (Eds.), *Handbook of counseling and psychotherapy with lesbian, gay, and bisexual clients.* Washington, D.C.: American Psychological Association.

Kellems, I. S., & Fassinger, R. E. (2003). The spiritual and religious lives of lesbians, gay men & bisexual individuals: Preliminary analyses. In R. Fassinger, *Results of the national gay and lesbian experiences study.* Symposium presented at the National Multicultural Conference and Summit III, Los Angeles, CA.

Kennet, J., Burgio, L., & Schulz, R. (2000). Interventions for in-home caregivers: A review of research 1990 to present. In Schulz, R. (Ed.), *Handbook on dementia caregiving: Evidence-based interventions for family caregivers* (pp. 61-125). New York: Springer.

Kimmel, D. (1995). Lesbians and gay men also grow old. In L. Bond, S. Cutler, & A. Grams (Eds.), *Promoting successful and productive aging* (pp. 289-303). Thousand Oaks, CA: Sage.

Levine, J. A., & Altman, C. (2002). Collaborating to support lesbian and gay caregivers for people with Alzheimer's. *Outword (Newsletter of the Lesbian & Gay Aging Issues Network), Winter.* San Francisco: American Society on Aging.

Lewinsohn, P. M., Muñoz, R. F., Youngren, M. A., & Zeiss, A. M. (1986). *Control your depression.* New York: Prentice Hall.

National Alliance for Caregiving and the American Association of Retired Persons (NAC/AARP). (2004). *Caregiving in the U.S.* Bethesda, MD: Author.

Moore, E. S. (1997). *Does your mama know? An anthology of Black lesbian coming out stories.* Decatur, GA: Red Bone Press.

Ory, M. G., Hoffman, R. R., Yee, J. L., Tennstedt, S., & Schulz, R. (1999). Prevalence and impact of caregiving: A detailed comparison between dementia and non-dementia caregivers. *The Gerontologist, 39,* 177-185.

Outword Online. (2000). San Jose, Calif.: Local needs assessment looks at LGBT elders. American Society on Aging's *Outword Online,* August, 2000.

Quam, J. K., & Whitford, G. S. (1992). Adaptation and age-related expectations of older gay and lesbian adults. *Gerontologist, 32,* 367-374.

REACH II Investigators (in press). Enhancing the quality of life of Hispanic/Latino, Black/African American, and White/Caucasian dementia caregivers. The REACH II Randomized Controlled Trial. *Annals of Internal Medicine.*

Reiter, B. (2003). New web-based outreach supports LGBT caregivers locally, nationally. *Outword, 9,* 1 & 6. San Francisco: American Society on Aging.

Roff, L., Burgio, L., Gitlin, L., Nichols, L., Chaplin, & Hardin, J. (2004). Positive aspects of Alzheimer's caregiving: The role of race. *Journals of Gerontology, 59B,* 185-190.

Ross, M. W., Paulsen, J. A., & Stalstrom, O. W. (1988). Homosexuality and mental health: A cross-cultural review. *Journal of Homosexuality, 15,* 131-152.

Schulz, R., & Beach, S. R. (1999). Caregiving as a risk factor for mortality: The caregiver health effects study. *JAMA, 282,* 2215-2219.

Schulz, R., O'Brien, A. T., Bookwala, J., & Fleissner, K. (1995). Psychiatric and physical morbidity effects of dementia caregiving: Prevalence, correlates, and causes. *The Gerontologist, 35,* 771-791.

Steffen, A. M. (2000). Anger management for dementia caregivers: A preliminary study using video and telephone interviews. *Behavior Therapy, 31,* 281-299.

Teri, L., Logsdon, R. G., & Uomoto, J. & McCurry, S. M. (1997). Behavioral treatment of depression in dementia patients: A controlled clinical trial. *Journal of Gerontology B: Psychological Science and Social Science, 52,* 159-166.

Thompson, L., Powers, D., Coon, D., Takagi, K., McKibbin, C., & Gallagher-Thompson, D. (2000). Older adults. In J. R. White & A. S. Freeman (Eds.), *Cognitive behavioral group therapy for specific problems and populations* (pp. 235-261). Washington, DC: American Psychological Association.

Weston, K. (1991). *Families we choose: Lesbians, gays, kinship.* New York: Columbia University Press.

Wight, R. G. (2002). AIDS caregiving stress among HIV-infected men. In B. J. Kramer & E. H. Thompson, Jr. (Eds.). *Men as caregivers: Theory, research, and service implications* (pp. 190-212). New York: Springer.

doi:10.1300/J041v18n03_07

Caregiving Research, Services, and Policies in Historically Marginalized Communities: Where Do We Go from Here?

Karen I. Fredriksen-Goldsen

Nancy R. Hooyman

SUMMARY. Future research, service interventions and policies must be responsive to the changing context of caregiving in this country and the increasing diversity in our society at large. This article examines the conceptual and methodological limitations that are inherent in the majority of the caregiving literature and outlines directions for future work on caregiving in marginalized communities, with a special emphasis on sexual orientation and gender identity. The article illustrates the importance of cultural variations and multiple identities as they relate to caregiving across diverse communities and explores ways to increase both theoretical and methodological rigor in future studies as well as ways to effectively access relatively hard to reach populations. As we move forward in caregiving research, services and policies, there is a critical need for increased attention to the societal context in which caregiving

Karen I. Fredriksen-Goldsen, PhD, is Associate Professor and Director, Institute for Multigenerational Health, School of Social Work, University of Washington, Seattle, WA.

Nancy R. Hooyman, PhD, is Endowed Gerontology Professor and Dean Emeritus, School of Social Work, University of Washington, Seattle, WA.

[Haworth co-indexing entry note]: "Caregiving Research, Services, and Policies in Historically Marginalized Communities: Where Do We Go from Here?" Fredriksen-Goldsen, Karen I., and Nancy R. Hooyman. Co-published simultaneously in *Journal of Gay & Lesbian Social Services* (The Haworth Press, Inc.) Vol. 18, No. 3/4, 2007, pp. 129-145; and: *Caregiving with Pride* (ed: Karen I. Fredriksen-Goldsen) The Haworth Press, Inc., 2007, pp. 129-145. Single or multiple copies of this article are available for a fee from The Haworth Document Delivery Service [1-800-HAWORTH, 9:00 a.m. - 5:00 p.m. (EST). E-mail address: docdelivery@haworthpress.com].

occurs–especially if we are to understand the realities of caregiving across marginalized and diverse communities. doi:10.1300/J041v18n03_08 *[Article copies available for a fee from The Haworth Document Delivery Service: 1-800-HAWORTH. E-mail address: <docdelivery@haworthpress.com> Website: <http://www.HaworthPress.com> © 2007 by The Haworth Press, Inc. All rights reserved.]*

KEYWORDS. Caregiving, family care, sexual orientation, gender identity, lesbian, gay, bisexual and transgender

INTRODUCTION

The social and political context in our country combined with long-standing cultural values form the societal backdrop for informal caregiving by family and friends. Our understanding of the range of caregiving experiences and types of effective informal and formal supports can be expanded by studying how historically disadvantaged groups manage the multiple demands of caregiving for their loved ones. The insights we glean from the study of caregiving within marginalized communities can deepen our understanding of the richness, diversity and resilience of people's lives across the life course.

Historically disadvantaged groups are conceptualized broadly in this paper to include those marginalized as a result of sexual orientation and gender identity as well as to include subgroups within these populations, defined by such factors as race and ethnicity, culture, and socio-economic status. In this paper we will specifically examine caregiving and care receiving among persons who self-identify as lesbian, gay, bisexual or transgender (LGBT), and address next steps in the following areas: (1) caregiving research; (2) services and intervention development; and (3) public policies.

This article begins by discussing the salience of multiple identities and cultural variations in understanding caregiving across such diverse communities. Next, we address ways to strengthen rigor in future research on informal care as it intersects with sexual orientation and gender identity. We emphasize several areas that have rarely been addressed in existing caregiving research: the need to develop effective means for reaching caregivers and care recipients in hidden populations, the critical role of the care relationship and interactions that may impact caregiving outcomes in terms of health and mental health, and the importance of theory development to guide future research. We highlight the salience of a life course approach that addresses the impact of culture, cohort, and individual life experience on caregiving as relationships and needs change over time. Next, we explore the need to develop services and test interventions aimed at assisting caregivers and care receivers in these communities. Lastly, we will scrutinize existing public policies and changes that are needed to improve caregiving outcomes within historically marginalized populations.

VARIATIONS IN LGBT COMMUNITIES

A growing number of practitioners and researchers are calling for the need to address caregiving within LGBT communities. Such critique assumes that the majority of caregiving research has been conducted with those only presumed to be heterosexual, since sexual orientation has been rarely identified and documented in most studies. Furthermore, in the caregiving research that does aim to address LGBT communities, the research findings tend to be extrapolated from one group and applied to others without attention to the potential variations that might exist across such historically marginalized groups.

To advance caregiving research, the constructs of sexual orientation and gender identity need to be more clearly articulated and understood.[1] While much of the current work tends to cluster LGBT issues, it is important to clearly define these constructs and then explore the similarities among these diverse groups as well as identify their unique needs and experiences. Although there is a small but growing body of literature on gay male and lesbian caregivers, there exists no significant representation of bisexual or transgender persons. Significant gender differences have been documented in the general caregiving literature, but more research is needed that explores the impact of gender roles and gender identity in the assumption of care responsibilities within LGBT communities.

With few exceptions, the majority of caregiving research has focused on Whites born in the United States, with relatively little known about informal care in racial and ethnic minority communities. There also has been limited attention to other cultural variations in caregiving, such as by geographic location or socio-economic status. For example, little is known about how varying cultural values and norms affect caregiving among LGBT racial and ethnic minorities.

Culture, defined broadly as a set of shared beliefs, values, behavioral norms, and practices that characterize a particular group of people who share a common identity (Hooyman & Kiyak, 2004), affects how caregiving is defined and experienced. Although rarely addressed in caregiving research, ethnic identity and degree of acculturation also tend to influence caregiving and care receiving experiences and outcomes. In a review of 59 articles published between 1980 and 2000, Dilworth-Anderson, Williams, and Gibson (2002) concluded that caregiving research needs to give more attention to issues of acculturation and cultural values, beliefs, and norms.

Existing research and conceptual models are inadequate for examining cultural variations in caregiving experiences within ethnic minority populations as well as among groups who have intersecting social identities in two or more historically marginalized communities. Future research will be strengthened by exploring experiences and outcomes among caregivers and care recipients with multiple identities based in the experience of marginalization. Such research would provide an important opportunity to explore experiences that may be distinctive to specific historically marginalized communities or that may cut across communities.

RESEARCH DIRECTIONS

Caregiving research within LGBT communities has important implications for a wide array of interdisciplinary fields, including public health, family studies, gerontology, sexuality, and gay and lesbian studies, to name a few. To move research forward, we will examine methodological advancements, such as innovations to reach hidden populations, theoretical and conceptual development, and the need to recognize the relational nature of caregiving.

Reaching Hidden Populations

A major limitation in existing research on LGBT caregiving lies in sample recruitment. Specifically, study participants have been largely recruited through snowball sampling techniques and convenience sampling, such as through lesbian/gay organizations. The research is also limited by homogeneity in age categories, since nearly all of the studies examine the life experiences of young adults; when specific to aging, studies have tended to focus on the youngest category of older adults. The result is that the current body of research primarily tends to reflect the lives of younger adults who are linked to gay and lesbian communities.

An important opportunity in future research is to address the distinctive methodological issues in studying hidden populations that exist in marginalized communities. To minimize the selection bias inherent in many of the existing studies, innovative sampling procedures are needed to strategically target relatively hidden members of historically marginalized communities who are not openly disclosing their identities, such as their sexual orientation or gender identity. In order to capture the potentially unique experiences of such diverse subsets within communities, future research would benefit from implementing methodological techniques for reaching individuals who are often reluctant to participate in research.

Sampling procedures to reach hidden populations have been developed, including target sampling (Watters & Biernacki, 1989; O'Connell, 2000), chain-referral, and respondent-driven sampling (Heckathorn, 1997). Although each of these techniques has individual strengths that need to be further explored in studies addressing marginalized communities, none of them alone deals with issues specific to reaching caregivers and care recipients within these groups. For example, the majority of such approaches have been designed to access stigmatized populations who, based on a behavior that draws them together, will be found congregating with one another (e.g., intravenous drug users who come together to use or sell drugs). However, among caregivers and care recipients, group identification alone does not necessarily provide a reason for congregating with others. One reason is that individuals who are providing care often do not define themselves as caregivers (Dobrof & Ebenstein, 2003/2004). Another factor is that the care recipient's functional impairment or the caregivers' time constraints created by multiple demands may decrease contact with others in their social network.

To address some of these constraints, the utilization of a mixed-method sampling approach could strengthen many studies by developing more representative sampling methods for hard-to-reach populations. In addition to the design of innovative sampling and recruitment strategies, the inclusion of questions on sexual orientation and gender identity into large national studies would help to expand our knowledge about these populations.

Theoretical and Conceptual Development

The literature base on caregiving in historically marginalized communities is limited by a general lack of theoretical and conceptual frameworks guiding the research. To date most studies of caregiving in LGBT communities utilize community-based needs assessments that lack firm theoretical grounding. Perhaps because of the lack of theoretical underpinnings of the research, the body of knowledge tends to represent more breadth than depth about caregiving within these diverse communities.

A life-course conceptual perspective to caregiving within historically marginalized populations provides a framework to examine the effects of age, cohort (generational difference), culture, and individual life experiences upon significant life transitions. Such a life course perspective could enhance understanding regarding whether adults across diverse communities have experienced similar or different life trajectories, and what impact specific risk and protective factors have had over the life course. Furthermore, such research enables investigators to explore the importance of other contextual issues, such as variations in culture, differing family context and structure, and cross-generational experiences in giving and receiving care. Generational issues related to cohort membership are likely to affect the caregiving and care receiving relationship and experience in marginalized communities, since significant generational differences exist in important areas such as identity development and disclosure.

Most caregiving research in the general population as well as in marginalized communities has been cross-sectional. Understanding how care roles and responsibilities change over time across the life course among marginalized populations requires longitudinal research designs. Longitudinal designs would allow researchers to examine more fully the causal relationships among the variables influencing caregiving within historically marginalized communities. In addition, they would capture not only the changes in care responsibilities that individuals experience over the course of their lives (including the care of children, disabled working-age adults, and elders) but also the ebb and flow of other life-cycle events over time (Fredriksen-Goldsen & Scharlach, 2001).

Caregiving: A Dyadic Process

To date, caregiving research has focused primarily on the individual caregiver and has not adequately addressed the often overlooked perspective of the care recipient and the importance of dyadic level processes and interactions that likely impact care relationships and outcomes. Similarly, few attempts have been made to understand how care experiences and outcomes vary by the nature of the care relationship. More research is needed to explore the interactional processes within the caregiver and care recipient relationship or dyad that may affect the extent to which the dyad may serve as a protective mechanism that moderates other risk factors in the caregiving experience.

Understanding the dyad as the unit of analysis is salient to examining caregiving within historically marginalized communities, since the type and duration of the care relationship may differ for dyads that are characterized by multiple identities and that experience discrimination and stigma. Among LGBT communities, formal services may be not be readily available, or may be underutilized because of actual and perceived barriers to accessing services. Understanding dyadic factors among such historically marginalized populations has implications for developing services and testing interventions to improve care outcomes.

SERVICE AND INTERVENTION DEVELOPMENT

Studies repeatedly demonstrate that negative physical and mental health outcomes exist among caregivers, but they less frequently identify whether services and interventions can alleviate those problems, especially within historically marginalized communities. Research directions that we have recommended will expand our understanding of historically disadvantaged care dyads' needs and experiences with formal services and of the internal, structural and policy barriers they face to service utilization; these data then can inform the development of interventions responsive to differences in sexual orientation and gender identity as well as cultural diversity.

As noted above, one internal barrier faced by most caregivers of dependents is their failure to identify themselves as performing essential care work and as deserving of services (Dobrof & Ebenstein. 2003/04). This is the case even when services such as respite, psycho-educational programs, adult day health, and social support groups are available. In addition to the lack of self identification, informal caregivers in general may not have the means to access services, such as the financial resources, transportation and respite needed to attend educational and social support groups. In many instances, caregivers in the general population are so busy with the multiple often conflicting demands of employment and their care work that they simply do not have the time to utilize such support services (Dilworth–Anderson, et al., 2002; Gartska, McCallion & Toseland, 2001; Mittelman, 2002).

These barriers that exist for the general population of caregivers of dependents are intensified for marginalized populations who face discrimination, are reluctant to disclose their sexual orientation to health care providers, are likely to have faced multiple losses of loved ones due to HIV/AIDS, and encounter legal and policy constraints from health and long-term care systems and the workplace. One of the primary structural barriers is that most service systems typically define informal caregivers as family members related by blood or marriage. Other systemic obstacles include being denied access to intensive care, medical records and decision-making about the care recipient, lack of legal protection, and insensitive treatment by information and referral systems that are the gateway to services (Brotman, Ryan, & Cormier, 2003; Cahill, South, & Spade, 2000; Coon & Burleson, 2006; Fredriksen, 1999). These discriminatory barriers, which increase the risk of negative health outcomes among LGBT caregiving dyads, are likely to be even greater in areas without established LGBT communities that provide social and instrumental support (Coon & Zeiss, 2003).

Interventions for caregivers generally have aimed to enhance the caregiver's ability to provide care and/or reduce the care recipient's needs for care. In the general caregiving literature, multi-level interventions encompassing psycho-education, support groups, and counseling that are targeted early on in the caregiving experience and are tailored to fit the care context are relatively effective in reducing negative caregiving outcomes (Schulz et al., 2002; Burgio et al., 2001; Burgio, Stevens Guy, Roth, & Haley, 2003; Toseland et al., 2001). Although some interventions have demonstrated clinically significant reductions in depressive symptoms among caregivers in the general population and delayed the care recipient's institutionalization (Schulz et al., 2002), most have targeted only the caregiver and have rarely taken into account the service needs of the dyad as a unit. Of greater concern is that the REACH project (Resources for Enhancing Alzheimer's Caregiver Health) (Schultz et al., 2002), which is the largest nationally-funded caregiving intervention, did not address any issues related to sexual orientation or gender identity and caregiving.

Intervention studies in LGBT communities are rare, although targeted social support interventions with HIV and AIDS caregivers and care recipients to enhance coping skills have been identified (McCausland, & Pakenham, 2003; Pakenham, Dadds, & Lennon, 2002). In addition, most interventions have not articulated how service providers' attitudes can be a significant barrier to effective service provision for marginalized populations.

We contend that multi-pronged service interventions with marginalized populations need to address not only the caregiving dyad, but also service providers' attitudes and behavior. Educational interventions with service providers are crucial because of the stigma, misinformation, and discrimination often exhibited by health and human service professionals toward care dyads in historically disadvantaged populations. Professionals need ongoing training and consultation to increase their understanding of the culture of marginalized populations and to ensure their competence in working with diverse historically disadvantaged groups (Coon, 2003; Coon & Zeiss, 2003). They also need to be informed about LGBT resources for care dyads and learn about marginalized population's experiences with such referrals. Inclusive language in brochures, websites, and other marketing of available services is critical to increasing access. In fact, we would argue that the service providers' attitudes and systemic barriers need to be addressed before developing dyadic-level interventions to address individual and interpersonal barriers to services.

As noted above, social support and educational interventions have been identified to reduce stress and enhance positive outcomes among caregivers generally. Yet support and psycho-education groups for dyads from marginalized populations need to take account of distinctive issues that differ from those faced by caregivers generally. These issues include experiences with discrimination based on sexual orientation or gender identity across the life course; biological family members' potential insensitivity or estrangement; greater reliance on partners and friends as caregivers; lack of workplace leave and other supports for these caregivers; and institutionalized heterosexism in health and long-term care settings that manifests in staff's discomfort with LGBT relationships. These barriers combined with lifelong experiences with discrimination may result in marginalized populations' unwillingness to disclose their sexual orientation or gender identity as the first step to accessing services. Service providers need early and explicitly to discuss strategies to protect confidentiality and privacy to reduce LGBT population's fears of self disclosure and reluctance to access services.

In such instances, on-line support groups or telephone counseling (individually or in groups) may be more effective at providing emotional support and problem solving than face to face meetings. These electronic forms of support also have the advantage of addressing time and geographic barriers. One example is a nationwide web-based LGBT Caregiver Discussion Group offered by the National Family Caregiver Alliance. However, individuals who are not internet-savvy or who are uncomfortable with on-line interactions may not utilize such electronic options.

Psycho-educational programs have also been determined to reduce stress among caregivers generally, especially when delivered in formats such as videos/DVDs, the internet, or manuals that are accessible on a 24 hour basis and at the caregivers' convenience. Such programs need to be modified, however, to include discussions of the barriers faced by marginalized populations in effectively managing their "outness" to service providers and in locating LGBT-competent services. Overall, just as providers must focus on providing culturally competent practice and policy, LGBT-competent interventions are needed across multiple levels to ensure support for both members of the caregiving dyad. Although such interventions with service providers and the individual care dyads are critical, policy advocacy is also essential, since marginalized populations face legal and systemic barriers to services.

PUBLIC POLICIES AND CAREGIVING

Given the current societal and political context, policy changes, such as reductions in Medicaid, are limiting services to all types of family caregivers. As is most often the case within the service sector, such changes, along with policies that are biased against LGBT caregivers, more negatively affect marginalized populations. For example, federal and state laws and institutional policies that provide benefits to assist caregiving families are generally biased against caregivers and care recipients in same-sex relationships, including the Family and Medical Leave benefits authorized by federal legislation, Social Security benefits, Medicaid spend-downs, and bereavement leave. In addition, the majority of laws that provide legal and economic protections for families exclude caregivers and care recipients in same-sex relationships, including nondiscrimination and state sanctioned marriage statutes.

Discrimination in Employment, Housing and Public Accommodation

Only 17 states and the District of Columbia have laws banning discrimination based on sexual orientation, and 100 municipalities in the other 33 states have local non-discrimination laws (Human Rights Campaign, 2003). Currently, only 8 states and the District of Columbia and 79 cities and counties have explicit transgender-inclusive anti-discrimination laws (National Gay and Lesbian Task Force, 2006).

The majority of the U.S. population has no protection in employment against discrimination due to sexual orientation or gender identity at either the federal, state or local level, and even more have no protection prohibiting discrimination in housing and public accommodations (Human Rights Campaign, 2003). Lack of protection from discrimination in employment leaves LGBT caregivers and their care recipients at risk for serious economic problems. Furthermore, since discrimination in housing and public accommodations is generally not prohibited, LGBT caregivers and their care recipients may be openly discriminated against in many housing arrangements and public accommodations, such as long-term care settings.

Legal Recognition of Primary Relationships

Currently, the public recognition of gay male and lesbian relationships is a hotly debated social issue: One state (Massachusetts) recognizes full marriage for same-sex couples. Legally sanctioned gay marriage represents a dramatic shift in pubic policy, and research is needed to ascertain the impact of such changing policies on those providing and receiving care. A few states such as Connecticut, New Jersey and Vermont allow civil unions; and, a few states and numerous city and county governments offer some sort of domestic partnership recognition. Same-sex marriages, civil unions and domestic partnerships, however, do not carry the benefit of federal recognition, which is necessary for Social Security and Medicaid benefits for partners. In addition, the majority of states have passed a version of the federal Defense of Marriage Act (DOMA), which explicitly bars recognition of same-sex couples (Cahill et al., 2002).

Legally recognized marriages bestow numerous rights, responsibilities, and benefits on married couples, many at the federal level. According to the General Accounting Office (GAO), there are more than 1,000 benefits, protections, and responsibilities that are automatically conferred to those who legally marry (Cahill et al., 2000). Among lesbian and gay male caregivers and their partners, legal recognition and protection are especially important in ensuring their ability to care for one another in the event of a health emergency or other crisis. Currently, if a lesbian or gay man becomes incapacitated and has not executed a legal durable power of attorney for health care, most state laws mandate that a legally married spouse or biological family members be appointed to manage affairs and make decisions, regardless of the disabled person's wishes (Epstein, 2003).

Family and Medical Leave Act

Under the federal Family and Medical Leave Act (FMLA) of 1993, employers with more than 50 employees are required to allow 12 weeks of unpaid leave during a 12-month period for employees to care for ill family members. Employers must continue health care coverage during such leaves and insure employees their jobs or equivalent positions on their return. Family leave has been endorsed by employees as the workplace policy most helpful to them in managing their family caregiving combined with their employment responsibilities (Fredriksen-Goldsen & Scharlach, 2001).

The FMLA provides unpaid leave only to an immediate family member (spouse, child, or parent) with a serious health condition and thus excludes those caring for same-sex partners or friends. Even when workplace specific family leave is available to same sex partners, employers' attitudes may nevertheless minimize the importance of caregiving responsibilities to LGBT partners or friends and be experienced as discriminatory (Coon & Burleson, 2006).

Supplemental Security Income (SSI) and Social Security Disability Insurance (SSDI)

While legally married couples and their children are entitled to Social Security survivor's benefits, same-sex couples are not (Cahill et al., 2000; Wenzel, 2002), and only in those states that recognize second-parent adoption can surviving children receive Social Security benefits (Cahill et al., 2000). Spousal benefits allow the surviving partner in a legally recognized marriage to collect the partner's benefit amount if that amount is greater than their own, based on their lifetime work history. For example, denial of spousal benefits to elder lesbian and gay male couples robs them of about $124 million per year in survivor's benefits, significantly impacting their economic well-being (Cahill et al., 2000).

The inequality of benefits for same-sex partners also extends to Social Security Disability Insurance. If a working-age adult becomes disabled, in addition to his or her own disability benefit, the legally married spouse also receives a monthly benefit of one-half of the monthly benefit of the disabled spouse. For a caregiver in a same-sex couple, there is no recognition of the relationship and, hence, no second benefit (Cahill et al., 2000).

Medicaid

Medicare will usually cover the first 100 days in a nursing home or skilled nursing facility needed for recuperation and rehabilitation after surgery or acute illness. However, Medicaid usually pays for long-term stays (more than 100 days) in nursing homes for disabled individuals who lack sufficient financial resources. The American Association of Retired Persons (AARP) estimates that in 1995 the average cost per day for nursing-home stays was $126, or about $46,000 per year (Kassner & Tucker, 1998).

For those who require nursing-home care but cannot afford it, Medicaid will pay for long-term care as well as needed home health care through the Medicaid "spend-down" program. The spend-down program has strict eligibility requirements for income and assets and is dependent on marital status. As of 1998, single individuals (those who are not legally married and hence those in same sex relationships) may only retain $2000 in assets, not counting home or car, in order to meet Medicaid spend-down requirements. Income allowances vary slightly from state to state, but generally if one is in a nursing home he or she may retain about $30 per month for personal expenses, or approximately $600 per month if an individual resides in the community (Washington Alaska Group Services [WAGSI], 2003). For federally recognized married couples, allowable assets and income vary from state to state, but generally a legally married couple residing in the community can retain between $1500 to $2300 per month. A significant disparity also exists in allowable assets, with legally married heterosexual couples allowed to retain approximately $18,000 to $90,000, depending on the state (WAGSI, 2003).

Another area in the Medicaid spend-down program that negatively impacts caregivers in same sex relationships is the estate recovery process. This program allows for the recovery of Medicaid expenditures from the estate of the deceased person, typically through the sale of the home or other assets. For heterosexual married couples, the state will generally not begin recovery proceedings (e.g., forced real property sale) from the estate until the surviving spouse has also died. This allows the survivor to remain in the home, without fear of impoverishment and/or homelessness. This benefit does not extend to non-married couples, meaning that upon the death of the loved one, the surviving partner and caregiver in a same sex relationship, may be forced to sell the home (if jointly owned) that they have shared and surrender half of the proceeds to the state (Cahill et al., 2000; WAGSI, 2003).

National Family Caregiver Support Program

In contrast to most employers, federal and state leave policies, the National Family Caregiver Support Program (NGCSP), passed by Congress in 2002, broadly defines informal or family caregivers as adult family members, friends or neighbors who provide care without pay and who usually have personal ties to the care recipient. The caregiver can be a "primary" or "secondary" caregiver, can provide full- or part-time help, and may live with the care recipient or separately. Under this definition, LGBT care dyads are able to access NFCSP services. However, caregivers must be age 60 and older and funding for NFCSP is relatively limited (National Association of State Units on Aging, 2003; HHS, 2004).

The NFCSP provides an example of the significance of defining caregiving broadly. Yet, most existing policies intended to help caregiving families in need clearly are biased against LGBT caregivers and their care recipients, further increasing their risk for marginalization, emotional stress, and economic problems. Given the current climate within which caregiving occurs, it is vital that advocacy efforts be aimed toward revising such biased public policies so that they provide the legal recognition necessary to protect LGBT caregivers and those receiving care.

Over the last decade there has been a significant reduction in publicly supported family care benefits. Currently, fragmented public policy initiatives exist to support caregivers and their loved ones, and even fewer are available to those providing and receiving care within LGBT communities. If we are to truly support family caregiving in this country, a comprehensive and coordinated public policy framework is desperately needed, including expanding family leave policies, advancing income support programs as well as developing a comprehensive long-term care system (Fredriksen-Goldsen & Scharlach, 2001). To increase equity and accessibility, it is imperative that public policy developments utilize broad definitions of caregivers and care receivers in order to recognize and support the pivotal role that same-sex partners and other extended family members and friends play in providing care across diverse communities.

CONCLUSION

Caregiving research, service interventions and workplace and public policies must be responsive to evolving family structures and care responsibilities within the context of increasing diversity across communities and the society at large. A number of emerging issues have the potential to substantially affect caregiving in the future, including the aging of the population, shifts in the nature of families who face growing economic pressures, and the societal context of caregiving. Most current family and caregiving programs and policies simply do not recognize the changing nature of the family and the important role of informal caregiving within historically marginalized communities.

Researchers and practitioners addressing caregiving will benefit from recognizing the extent of care that is provided in historically disadvantaged communities, including those marginalized as a result of sexual orientation and gender identity. Furthermore, as we move forward in research, service and policy development it is critical to differentiate between strategies to create caregiving supports that are adaptations to existing structures and norms versus efforts to change them so they are truly inclusive of the diverse arrangements and needs of all families (Fredriksen-Goldsen & Scharlach, 2001). Ultimately, efforts will need to be directed at changing social norms and policies that support the mutual well-being of LGBT caregivers and care recipients within the larger societal context.

NOTE

1. Sexual orientation reflects interpersonal attractions and the desires and feelings involved (Lorber, 1994), including those attracted emotionally and sexually to a different sex (heterosexuals), one's one sex (lesbians and gay males), and those attracted emotionally and sexually to both males and females (bisexuals). Gender identity refers to a person's internal, deeply felt sense of being either male or female, or other. Transgender is an umbrella term referring to those who identify as other than their biological sex.

REFERENCES

Brotman, S., Ryan, B., & Cormier, R. (2003). The health and social service needs of gay and lesbian elders and their families in Canada. *The Gerontologist, 43*(2), 192-202.

Burgio, L., Lichstein, K. L., Nichols, L., Czaja, S., Gallagher-Thompson, D., Bourgeois, M., et al. (2001). Judging outcomes in psychosocial interventions for dementia caregivers: The problem of treatment implementation. *Gerontologist, 41,* 481-489.

Burgio, L., Stevens, A., Guy, D., Roth, D. L & Haley, W. E. (2003). Impact of two psychosocial interventions on white and African American family caregivers of individuals with dementia. *The Gerontologist, 43*, 568-581.

Cahill, S., Ellen, M., & Tobias, S. (2002). *Family Policy: Issues affecting gay, lesbian, bisexual, and transgender families.* New York: The Policy Institute of the Gay and Lesbian Task Force.

Cahill, S., South, K., & Spade, J. (2000). How aging policy frameworks can benefit GLBT elders. Outing age. *Public policy issues affecting gay, lesbian, bisexual and transgender elders.* New York: The Policy Institute of the National Gay and Lesbian Task Force, 36-63.

Coon, D. W. (2003). *Lesbian, gay, bisexual and transgender (LGBT) issues and family caregiving.* San Francisco, CA: Family Caregiver Alliance, National Center on Caregiving.

Coon, D. W. & Burleson, M. H. (2006). Working with gay, lesbian, bisexual, and transgender families. In Yeo, G. & Gallagher-Thompson, D. (Eds.) *Ethnicity and the Dementias (2nd ed.)* (pp. 343-358). New York: Routledge Taylor & Francis Group.

Coon, D. W., & Zeiss, L. M. (2003). Caregiving for families we choose: Intervention issues with LGBT caregivers. In D. W. Coon, D. Gallagher-Thompson, & L. Thompson (Eds.) *Innovative interventions to reduce dementia caregiver distress: A clinical guide* (pp. 267-295). New York: Springer.

Department of Health and Human Services, (2004) *The Older Americans Act: National Family Caregiver Support Program. Compassion in action.* Washington, D.C.: Administration on Aging.

Dilworth-Anderson, P., Williams, I. C. & Gibson, B. E. (2002). Issues of race, ethnicity, and culture in caregiving research: A 20-year review (1980-2000). *Gerontologist, 42*(2), 237-272.

Dobrof, J., & Ebenstein, H. (2003/2004). Family caregiver self-identification: Implications for healthcare and social service professionals. *Generations, 27*(4), 33-38.

Epstein, A. (2003, December 19) Gay basics: Partner medical rights documentation. *Gay Financial News.*

Fredriksen, K. I. (1999). Family caregiving responsibilities among lesbians and gay men. *Social Work, 44*(2), 142-155.

Fredriksen-Goldsen, K. I., & Scharlach, A. E. (2001). *Families and work: New directions in the twenty-first century.* New York: Oxford University Press.

Gartska, T., McCallion, P., & Toseland, R. (2001). Using support groups to improve caregiver health. In M. L. Hummert and J. F. Nussbaum (Eds.), *Aging, communication and health.* Mahwah, NJ: Lawrence Erlbaum Associates.

Heckathorn, D. (1997). Respondent-driven sampling: A new approach to the study of hidden populations. *Social Problems, 44*(2), 174-199.

Hooyman, N. R., & Kiyak, A. H. (2004). *Social gerontology: A multidisciplinary perspective (7th Ed.).* Boston: Allyn and Bacon.

Kassner, E., & Tucker, N. G. (1998). *Medicaid and long-term care for older people.* Washington, DC: Public Policy Institute, American Association of Retired Persons.

Lorber, J. (1994). *Paradoxes of Gender.* New Haven, CT: Yale University Press.

McCausland, J., & Pakenham, K. I. (2003). Investigation of the benefits of HIV/AIDS caregiving and relations among caregiving adjustment, benefit finding, and stress and coping variables. *AIDS Care, 15*(6), 853-869.

Mittelman, M. S. (2002). Family caregiving for people with Alzheimer's disease: Results of the NYU Spouse Caregiver Intervention Study. *Generations, 3*, 104-106.

National Association of State Units on Aging (NASUA). (2003).*The aging network implements the National Family Caregiver Support Program.* Washington, D.C.: Administration on Aging.

National Gay & Lesbian Taskforce (March, 2006) *Jurisdictions with explicitly transgender-inclusive anti-discrimination laws.* Washington, D.C. Author.

O'Connell, A. (2000). Sampling for evaluation: Issues and strategies for community-based HIV prevention programs. *Evaluation & the Health Professions, 23*(2), 212-234.

Pakenham, K., Dadds, M., & Lennon, H. (2002). The efficacy of a psychosocial intervention for HIV/AIDS caregiving dyads and individual caregivers: A controlled treatment outcome study. *AIDS Care, 14*(6), 731-750.

Schulz, R., O'Brien, A., Czaaja, S., Ory, M., Norris, R., Martire, L. M., et al. (2002). Dementia caregiver intervention research: In search of clinical significance. *Gerontologist, 42,* 589-602.

Toseland, R., McCallion, P., Smith, T., Huck, S., Bourgeois, P., & Garstka, T. (2001). Health education group for caregivers in an HMO. *Journal of Clinical Psychology, 57,* 551-570.

Washington Alaska Group Services. (2003). Medicaid. Retreived December 18, 2003 from http://www.wagsltc.com/medicaid/.

Watters, J. K., & Biernacki, P. (1989). Target sampling: Options for studying hidden populations. *Social Problems, 36*(4), 416-431.

Wenzel, H. V. (2002). *Fact sheet: Legal issues of LGBT caregivers* (Fact Sheet). San Francisco, CA: Family Caregiver Alliance.

doi:10.1300/J041v18n03_08

Index

Abuse, transgender people and, 105
Activities of caregiving, 44-46,45*t*
Adultery, as punishable sex act, 94-95
Age
    caregiver distress and, 59,61-62,64*t*
    comparisons of
        caregivers/recipients, 27*t*
    demographics of LGBT caregivers,
        42*t*
    LGBT community and, 4
    as predictor of willingness to
        provide caregiving, 30*t*
    resilience and, 56*f*,57
Aging population
    as caregivers. *see* Caregiving
    caregiving in Native communities
        and, 76
    comparisons of
        caregivers/recipients, 27*t*
    discrimination and, 103
    discussion and, 29-35
    increase in, 2
    predictors of willingness to provide
        caregiving, 30*t*
    resilience and, 9
    survey design/methodology and,
        20-25
    survey introduction and, 16-20
    survey results and, 26-29
    survey summary and, 15-16
    transgender people and, 102-104
AIDS. *see* HIV/AIDS
American Indian LGBT community.
    see Two-spirit people
Americans with Disabilities Act,
    transgender people and, 99

Anal gonorrhea, as threat for older
    LGBT adults, 30
Antiretroviral therapy, HIV/AIDS and,
    54
Anxiety, two-spirit people and, 76-77
ART. *see* Antiretroviral therapy
Attack (gay-related), past caregiving
    experiences and, 22

Behavioral techniques, SURE 2 and,
    117-118,120-121
Berdache, 78
Bias. *see* Discrimination
Blood cell count, transgender people
    and, 98
Blood clots, transgender people and,
    99
Bone density, transgender people and,
    98-99
Burden
    comparisons of
        caregivers/recipients, 27*t*
    correlation matrix of key variables,
        47*t*
    hierarchical multiple regression of
        caregiver burden for LGB
        family of origin/choice
        caregivers, 48*t*
    as predictor of willingness to
        provide caregiving, 30*t*
    predictors of, 46-48
    as a result of caregiving, 19,24
    support and. *see* Informal support
    two-spirit people and, 76-77,87-88

T - #0575 - 101024 - C0 - 212/152/9 - PB - 9781560237594 - Gloss Lamination